DO AS I SAY,
NOT WHO I DID.

DO AS
I SAY,
NOT
WHO
I DID.

HONEST ADVICE ON HOOKUPS
AND RELATIONSHIPS IN COLLEGE

ALI DRUCKER

THE EXPERIMENT
NEW YORK

The Experiment, LLC
220 East 23rd Street, Suite 600
New York, NY 10010-4658
theexperimentpublishing.com

This book contains the opinions and ideas of its author. It is sold with the understanding that the author and publisher are not rendering personal professional services. The author and publisher specifically disclaim all responsibility for any liability, loss, or risk—personal or otherwise—that is incurred as a consequence, directly or indirectly, of the use and application of any of the contents of this book.

THE EXPERIMENT and its colophon are registered trademarks of The Experiment, LLC. Many of the designations used by manufacturers and sellers to distinguish their products are claimed as trademarks. Where those designations appear in this book and The Experiment was aware of a trademark claim, the designations have been capitalized. The Experiment's books are available at special discounts when purchased in bulk for premiums and sales promotions as well as for fundraising or educational use. For details, contact us at info@ theexperimentpublishing.com.

Library of Congress Cataloging-in-Publication Data available upon request

ISBN 978-1-61519-796-5
Ebook ISBN 978-1-61519-797-2

Jacket design by Erin Seaward-Hiatt
Text design by Beth Bugler
Author photograph by Matt Martin

Manufactured in the United States of America

First printing April 2022
10 9 8 7 6 5 4 3 2 1

Some names and identifying details have been combined or changed to protect the privacy of individuals.

To all those discovering
what you want and learning
how to ask for it.

To you.

Contents

Orientation Starts Now

It was sophomore year of college and I was lying on my back, half naked, when I noticed something starting to sting, and then, slowly, burn. After I gently tapped my partner on the shoulder, he popped up from between my legs and asked what was wrong. I was about to say, "I'm not sure," when I noticed to my utter horror there was an Altoid mint still in his mouth. Equal parts mortified and traumatized, I ran out of my dorm and into the shower, rinsing the residue of winter-fresh mint out of my vagina.

And then, of course, I immediately went to the dining hall and told all my friends, warning them of my urban-legend-esque hookup disaster that had turned all too real.

That moment was perhaps the genesis of this book, in its own odd way. Not because I think the world needs informing about the perils of after-dinner mints, but because there are far too few resources to prepare us for the scenarios we have no idea we might face when it comes to our intimate lives. Simply put, the purpose of this book is to give practical advice for an impractical time: college.

In the first two months after arriving at school, I had already hooked up with three guys who lived on my dorm floor. That's not one, not two, but three daily opportunities to awkwardly bump into someone who had seen me naked as I scurried, shower cap–clad, to the bathroom. By my second year, I knowingly made out with my friend's crush in front of her at a party. I told my boyfriend I loved him while high on mushrooms. My friends kept track of the number of shots they'd taken by marking horizontal slashes on their forearms with a marker; I kept track of all my sexual partners in an iPhone note because I was scared I'd forget.

These kinds of impulsive antics are what college is about. But like many of my peers, I'd had only basic sex ed at my suburban high school, and though I arrived on campus with some experience (assuming you consider a few sessions of awkward, fumbling sex that resulted in approximately zero orgasms "experience"), I felt completely in the dark about the difference between "antic" and "unnecessary risk." And things didn't clear up anytime soon.

After a whole bunch of trial and error, I learned how to balance my newfound social freedom with the real reason I came to college in the first place (learning, duh). But grasping those lessons didn't always feel good: Having to ask your friend for the Geology notes because you and your boyfriend slept through class together doesn't exactly make you feel like you're getting the most out of school. I'd often wished I had the benefit of some older, wiser, cooler, nonjudgmental voices to shepherd me along—and maybe even help me make smarter decisions, like perhaps not volunteering to be the model for the clue "cheese whiz bikini" on an R-rated campus scavenger hunt. So I've written the book I wish I'd had when I was in school.

In these pages you will find straightforward, unflinchingly honest, and research-backed sex and dating advice from myself and experts in the field of sexuality whom I consulted, with the ultimate goal of helping you develop a healthy sex life as you prepare for and navigate the most exciting—and often the most confusing—years of your life. So enjoy the education. It is college, after all.

Heads-up: This book contains frank discussions about unwanted sexual contact throughout.

1.

You Don't Owe Anyone Sex

Giving, Getting, and Withdrawing Consent

"**I** don't know why this is happening to me," Jacob said, pulling on his boxers and conveniently avoiding eye contact. "I've been with girls much hotter than you." Instantly stung, I flushed a shade of red impossible to see under the blue glow of his Mac-Book. You'll never forget where you were the first time a guy blames you for his erectile dysfunction. I sure as hell can't. And I've tried.

I was one week into my first semester of college and didn't know why someone who was complimenting me hours ago would be insulting me now. But instead of throwing off the twin extra-long sheets and storming out of his dorm, I stayed and listened to him explain why his lack of an erection was my fault. I did eventually leave, exhausted by both his placement of me on the spectrum of his sexual partners' hotness and from feigning enthusiasm for his soft boner in my mouth, but more than a decade later that memory haunts me more than the bangs I cut myself four days before my freshman year.

I wouldn't realize why until much later, but even in the moment I knew something felt off. This wasn't how I thought college would be. These four years, bursting with parties, new friends, and fun hookups, were supposed to save me from a high school experience that had left me feeling broken and insecure. But is this what salvation looked like? Sneaking through the common room with lingerie under my zip-up hoodie for sex with someone who was using me to coax confidence back into his sad, shy penis? It didn't seem fair, but I felt powerless to object.

And maybe his cruel joke of a rejection hurt so much precisely because I felt powerless. Before I left for my first year of college, I spent an awkward summer in therapy trying to make sense of the fact that I suddenly had no friends. I had never been popular in school. (Fun fact: The one and only time I ran for student council, my classmates started chanting my opponent's name at me when I walked into homeroom.) After high school graduation, though, even my small social circle had unwound. Every single friend I had considered close just stopped talking to me en masse. I couldn't understand it, but deep in my anxious bones I figured it must have been my fault and they'd just grown tired of having me around. With no explanation, their invitations and messages simply stopped coming. To this day I have never found out why. Weekend sleepovers and marathon messaging gave way to Friday nights at home with my parents, when I'd fantasize about the new life I'd start in college. I was the only person I knew who didn't feel a whiff of sentimentality about leaving my hometown; I couldn't wait to get away.

Helping to build my anticipation were the hours I logged trolling all the "Incoming Freshman" Facebook groups to get a look at my future friends and, I'd hoped, guys who I could convince via a series of hook-ups to eventually date me. I spent so much time glued to my family's desktop computer that I even discovered a way to sort people's profiles by sex, age, and relationship status. I called it the Boy Catalog (yes, I actually said those words out loud to people!), and I would click through to build a mental Rolodex of every available guy in both my class and future dorm. That's where I first spotted Jacob. He was a sophomore on the hockey team, and in his photos he rocked a scruffy beard—a rarity in the dating pool when you're eighteen.

So, fresh off my Summer of Social Rejection, when I bumped into Jacob the first week of classes and he smiled at me, I felt I had somehow willed this blessing into existence. All my late-night wishing and clicking had brought A Real-Life Hot Man into my life. Suddenly, it didn't matter anymore who had rejected me in my past. I had the sort-of affection of a cute older guy, and that had to count for something. Sure, he playfully put me down in a way that kind of made me feel bad but, I thought, this only proved his effortless coolness. And that is exactly how you wind up staying in bed with a man who implies that you're not very pretty and expects it to turn you on. Raw trauma and internet stalking make for one potent cocktail of bad decisions.

When, late one night, Jacob asked me to come to his room for the first time, it didn't matter that he seemed just a bit creepier than my projected ideal of him constructed from carefree and well-tanned Facebook photos. He wanted to spend time with me, a girl who came to college in Converse sneakers covered in Sharpie-scrawled Green Day lyrics; a girl who would gladly tell you why Franz Kafka was her favorite writer; a girl who hadn't had a friend to confide in for months. We all come into relationships with unique vulnerabilities, and whether or not we realize it, those vulnerabilities can affect the way we're able to communicate what we really want. Jacob's attention made me feel valuable to both myself and others for the first time in a long while. I was conflicted, but ultimately it felt like I had no choice but to push aside my momentary doubts. I had wanted this, right? So how could I say no?

It turns out I couldn't, even when he started to show his true colors beneath the brightly hued hockey jersey. The whole you're-not-that-hot-so-I-don't-know-why-my-penis-is-intimidated-by-you thing didn't break me at first, but I continued to show up eager at his dorm and would then leave dejected. Each time, I was giving more and more of myself away. The idea of withdrawing my consent to sleep with him—taking it all back and walking away—felt impossible. I clung blindly to the notion that if I held up my end of the bargain (showing up whenever he texted) maybe he'd eventually start caring if I was having fun. It took a final blow to my self-esteem to snap some sense into place. After a few weeks, he flat-out said he didn't want any of his teammates to know we were hooking up, and that I should "keep it quiet." Those words made me not just realize but actually accept that he was only looking for quick and easy sex, wherein he wouldn't have to be accountable to anyone else's feelings. It should have been a red flag that basically every time we had sex I was counting down the minutes until it was over, but the newness and excitement of it all had left me colorblind.

Finally deciding I wanted to stop seeing him was relatively easy; dealing with the fallout of my own self-flagellation was much harder. I felt embarrassed, and something more sinister: guilt. Shouldn't I have seen this coming? How could I have picked my partners so poorly? While it's true that there's some correlation[1] between the low self-esteem I was suffering from and risky sexual behavior, more than anything else I wish I could go back in time, shake my eighteen-year-old self, and tell her that male shittiness is not your fault, there's nothing you did to deserve it, and there's literally no one to whom you owe sex. And while my past self is busy time traveling, I'd kindly ask her to make a detour and deliver to Jacob a robust "fuck you," and let him know I have since had sex with lots of guys hotter than him, thanks very much.

Still, it eats away at me that I kept making weekly visits to his dorm for longer than I should have, even after he shook my already fragile sense of self-worth. I hadn't had many partners at that point and didn't know that I could demand better—I didn't even know what "better" would look like—but I *did*

> ## How could I say no now if I'd said yes before?

know that the sex itself was forgettable and even though he often hurt my feelings, I stuck around anyway.

Looking back, I know I fully consented to sex with Jacob before we started having it. But each and every time, halfway through, I *wished* I hadn't. I wanted to take it back but was stopped by guilt and embarrassment. How could I say no now if I'd said yes before? What would he tell other guys about me? It's not surprising that I didn't know how to stop what had already started: I had absolutely no established protocol to extricate myself from a situation that had become unpleasant. Thankfully, today the nuances of consent are more widely discussed than they were when I was bouncing between Jacob (who mistook me, a real-life human woman, for a Viagra prescription) and Carter (who got pouty when I told him I didn't want to have anal sex and neglected to disclose that he was also sleeping with two other women on my dorm floor). Of course, just because people are talking more about consent today doesn't mean everyone is really listening. And even when we're listening, we still don't always understand.

To figure out what I could have done differently, I'd have to go back to the basics. So I did.

CONSENT 101

Definitions and Misconceptions

Here it is: Consent is an agreement between sexual partners that you're both on board with what's about to happen between you; that agreement is reassessed each time someone wants to try something new on an ongoing basis. Vanessa Marin, a California-based sex therapist I spoke with, puts it something like this: "Consent is saying 'yes' to a sexual situation, but more importantly, feeling *good* about that yes." (If you've heard the term "*enthusiastic* consent," that's what it means.) You're not saying yes because you're afraid of what will happen if you don't, or because you're worried someone will think you're a prude, or because you're hoping this will win them over and lead to a relationship. You're saying yes because the things that are happening make you and your body feel good.

It's a little ironic that the most important word when it comes to healthy sex is the least sexy-sounding, like you're begrudgingly signing your rights away to have some unpleasant medical procedure performed. And that's where a lot of us start to lose the threads of a relatively straightforward idea, both honestly and in bad faith. Sabrina, nineteen, who just finished her first year at the University of Jacksonville in Florida, told me that she gives consent by agreeing to go home with a guy—her signal that she wants to be intimate with him. But in what ways? How do you let someone know which specific things you're down for? Sabrina didn't have a clear answer. She, like all the young women I spoke to in my research on this topic, gets it in theory: No one should be doing things in bed they don't want to do. But in practice, it's more complicated.

One popular misconception about consent goes back to the clinical, almost nerdiness of the word. Sabrina admitted it's a phrase that's been tossed around so much it's become a little bit of a joke, and she and her friends tease one another with calls of "Oh, ya gotta consent!" before a hookup, in the same way you'd tease your mom if she reminded you to grab a jacket before you left the house on a 70-degree day. In this way, a foundational aspect of sex has become a punchline. People critiquing the idea in bad faith use that to their advantage.

I keep thinking about an episode of *The Unbreakable Kimmy Schmidt*, Tina Fey and Robert Carlock's comedy starring Ellie Kemper. In season three, Kimmy, who attends Columbia University, starts flirting with a guy at a party. Then he turns to her, whips out paper and pen, and requests that they review and sign each other's sexual consent forms. It's played for laughs, though it's difficult to tell if the show's creators are mocking younger generations who actually give a shit about making sure they're not assaulting someone, or if they're critiquing the notion that consent needs to be so dramatic. Either way, it's a fair representation of how people deem discussions of consent unnecessary, even silly. And look, if you want to write down the things you're into before sleeping with someone new, then great! That could work really well for you! But it's certainly not an immovable requirement to getting someone's consent, and it's definitely not the only way to do so. When people characterize the getting and giving of consent like an accountant itemizing your taxes, pausing to consult their calculator at every new line, they're minimizing what's really at play: making sure you're not taking advantage of someone, or being taken advantage of.

Of course, some of the confusion around the term is valid. How could we possibly be expected to understand a concept so rarely taught in schools? Right now, only eight states[2] require sex-ed classes to teach lessons about consent. So, to Sabrina's point, you've agreed to go home with someone. You know something is going to happen. What now?

Here's another commonly misunderstood aspect of consent: Consent is fluid in that it needs to be reestablished with each new sexual act. Just because you're into a hot make-out session doesn't mean someone can then stick their hand down your pants if you haven't indicated you'd be into that, too. I like to think about it like buying a plane ticket. If I have an economy boarding pass, it doesn't mean I can just walk into first class and sit down simply because there's an empty seat. It also doesn't mean I can ride every single flight from now on.

And that's one of the first places I went wrong with Jacob, and too many others after him. Marin acknowledges it's a common misconception that consent is like a blank check that the initiator gets to fill in. "I think a lot of people do think that if you say yes to something, you're saying yes to anything or committing to sticking something through regardless of what your experience was like in the moment," she explains. But that couldn't be further from the truth.

CONSENT 201

Giving and Getting

Okay, you're with someone you like, and things seem to be turning physical. So how do you give or get consent? Often, hookups will start with a kiss. Ideally, the person initiating the kiss will ask first. You might just keep making out, or you may decide you want to try something new. If you and your partner are both turned on and they're doing something you like, you can indicate your consent in a number of nonverbal ways: pulling your partner in for a deeper kiss, moaning (think a throaty "mmmm!" rather than "oooaAAAHHHhhh!"), wrapping your legs around them, you name it. But for a few reasons we'll get into later, verbal consent is often more helpful. One way to have these conversations is to weave them seamlessly into the types of hot whisperings you'd want to hear in bed anyway. "We have this idea that having to communicate during sex is weird or awkward or it's a sign there's no chemistry," Vanessa Marin explains. "I think it's not only crucial for having a happy

Consent is fluid in that it needs to be reestablished with each new sexual act.

and healthy sex life, but it can also be really sexy in the moment."

Megan, twenty, who attends a small college in the Northeast, agrees. When she got to campus, she was shocked by how little some of her peers communicated about sex. She vividly recalls having sex with a guy she met early on in her first semester. After they slept together, he told her, "Oh, that was my first time." Surprised, Megan asked, "Your first time doing what?" And while it's obviously up to the individual whether or not they want to disclose such information, the admission that it was his first time having sex still made Megan feel a bit guilty and uncomfortable. She realized just how little they had spoken before hooking up; at the very least, she would have wanted to be more present, communicative, and supportive of him if she had known.

Since then, her pre-sex communication has improved, especially where consent is concerned. Now, she'll directly ask, "Oh, do you want to have sex?" And then to work out specifically what's on the table, she'll say, "Tell me what you want." As she explains it, "I feel like that's a good one because we could still be in the 'mood,' but it's very explicitly asking you what you want here." There's still a lot of imbalance in the system, though. Megan acknowledges that people are more likely to be attuned to the dynamics of consent when they're trying something new or potentially out of someone's comfort zone—which is important, but these conversations should really be happening across the board. She's also found that most of her male partners will ask a cursory question or two at the start, but don't check in on an ongoing basis. It shouldn't be a woman's job to educate men

Further proof that sex is nothing like the movies: You should feel free to talk during the good parts.

on how to have these conversations. It is, however, to our society's collective benefit if as many people as possible start modeling consensual, active question asking and answering when it comes to sex.

With that in mind, here are some places to start. Because (A) dirty talking is hard, and (B) no one will ever know you stole these from me. Please don't show this to your mom.

A nonexhaustive list of what you can say or ask to give and get consent

"I want your tongue in between my thighs, will you do that for me, baby?"

"I can't wait to feel your [insert your favorite euphemism for penis here!] inside me."

"Can I taste your [insert body part here]?"

"I've been thinking all day it would be so hot if we [insert sex thing here]."

"I want to put my lips on every part of your body. Where should I put them first?"

"I want you to start kissing my neck and work your way down. Don't stop until you want to."

"Have you ever fantasized about [insert sex thing you want to try here]?"

"I want to [insert sex thing here] in every inch of this room. Where should we start?"

What these phrases have in common is that they either signify intent (so no one has a random sex act sprung on them), pose questions, or open up space for a partner to say no or offer up an alternative. Plus, they're kind of sexy.

But not everyone cares if getting consent sounds hot. Maggie, nineteen, a rising junior at Manhattan College, is one of those people. The first time she had sex, it was coerced. Her high school boyfriend, according to Maggie, constantly wore her down by telling her she wasn't good enough for him and she should have been doing more to please him. "He was very manipulative and abusive, and I felt like if I didn't do what he wanted he would be upset with me," Maggie says. But Maggie didn't understand that she ultimately said yes under duress—not a true yes at all—until her second semester of freshman year when she took a course all about the interplay of sex and violence, especially as it's portrayed in the media. With her eyes newly opened to these issues, she found her current boyfriend, who's a breath of fresh air. "He'll ask to do anything, even hold my hand or walk me to my dorm, and I didn't realize that's what I needed. It just makes me feel so much more comfortable knowing that I have a say in what's going on."

When they're having sex, her boyfriend takes a similar approach and asks before each new act. And it doesn't kill the mood at all. "It's like, *Wow, he actually cares what I want.* That means a lot to me and it's a turn-on for me, actually."

Further proof that sex is nothing like the movies: You should feel free to talk during the good parts.

The Other G-Spot: Guilt

The unique environment of college can impact consent in a number of upsetting ways (think: lots of people who don't know one another well coming together at boozed-up parties). No one knows this better than Natalie, twenty, a rising junior at a small university in Pennsylvania. Natalie explained to me that if you're under twenty-one, the only way to enjoy the nightlife at her school is to go to frat parties, because they have the booze. That's pretty standard fare for many schools with Greek life, but what she told me next is not. In order to attend one of those parties, you have to text a fraternity brother. Then, according to Natalie, they'll look you up and decide if you're attractive enough to come. Once that's settled, they'll assign a brother to come pick you up in his car and escort you into the party. When she started telling me this, I interrupted her. "Wait, even if you're invited? They have to actually come get you?"

"Oh yeah, they'll turn you away. You can't Uber there. You can't walk," Natalie explained. This is all in a bid to reduce unwanted attention from the cops, according to the fraternity brothers. Fewer cars and less foot traffic help them keep a low profile. "It's horrible," she admitted. "But the worst part is that to leave the party, you also have to be escorted. So you have to wait on a line to leave. And sometimes that can be, like, an hour wait." My jaw dropped. College truly is a minefield when it comes to navigating these issues with any sort of confidence or clarity. These fraternities have essentially designed a way to hold women captive at their parties. First, the selection process ensures that girls feel lucky, even flattered, just to be invited through the doors. Then, they're completely beholden to those same guys for the rest of the night if they want to leave. Discouraging girls from leaving may be the point. Natalie herself has had nights at these parties when she wanted to go, took one look at the long line of guests awaiting a ride, then went right back inside. It's this exact environment—feeling grateful to be there and wary of pissing off your hosts—that makes consent so challenging on campus.

Natalie told me about a party where she was on the dance floor, making out with a frat brother. She was having a great time and told me the interaction was totally consensual. But then he cornered her into a secluded area of the house and started to take his pants off in front of her. She froze, rebuffed him, and walked away. But that memory stuck with her. "This is going to sound so bad," she prepped me. "And this was me two years ago, so I've had time to reflect on this. But in the moment, I think I felt just embarrassed. I felt guilty that I didn't do anything. As if I had owed him that, and I obviously did not."

What might give Natalie an idea like that? Well, a lot of factors, like a tightly engineered party that makes girls sitting ducks—not to mention our socialization of boys and girls from a young age, which is another good place to start. It's no secret that girl toys and boy toys are still markedly different: Boys get trucks and blocks; girls get dolls and pretend kitchens. The former emphasizes active play and problem solving, the latter passive play and nurturing. I'm generalizing here, and many companies have branched out with more inclusive offerings, but the play divide still remains. This kind of expectation and bias follows kids as they grow up; studies show teachers are more likely to invest time in talking to boys and more likely to interrupt girls in the classroom. Add up a lifetime of these stereotypes and microaggressions and women can become socialized to be accommodating, kind, and caretakers of other people's feelings—whether we realize it or not. Fast-forward, and if a woman is experiencing something in bed that she doesn't really like, it can be a lot harder to speak up about it—and harder still to plainly state "I don't consent to this."

The guilt of not wanting to hurt our partner's feelings is a palpable force. Take my friend Lauren, now twenty-nine. In our sophomore year of college, Lauren was hooking up with a guy she was really into. When he stopped returning her texts, she was distraught. One night a couple of weeks later, we all went to a house party at the home of Lauren's exhookup. And, still raw from some tender hurt feelings, Lauren started flirting with her ex's housemate. It was innocent enough. She was trying to get back out there, to boost her confidence, and sure, it didn't hurt that another guy was paying attention to her in front of the ex who had ghosted her. Let it be said: Sometimes you want to flirt for flirting's own sake, and that is fine. What happened next wasn't. As the night started winding down and people started leaving, Lauren noticed the way her ex's housemate was looking at her. She could tell from the way he was intently meeting her gaze that he expected they were going to hook up.

"It felt like I already agreed to hook up with him, like it was kind of a social contract that *this* is where this is going. And by flirting, I'm agreeing, yes, I will hook up with you tonight," she explained to me, recalling the night years later. But she hadn't wanted the night to go there. I asked her why she didn't feel like she could tear up that social contract, and she rattled off a list of reasons that sounded all too familiar. We were all in the same circle of friends; it would be awkward the next day; she had been flirting with him earlier; we had been drinking their beer at their house. It goes on. She hadn't done anything wrong, but she felt all that guilt mounting.

> "When you're in a traumatic situation, it's not just fight or flight. It's fight, flight, or freeze."

Lauren says she knew she had flirted with him and consented to his touching her back, but she didn't want the hookup that eventually followed. She just didn't know how to draw the line of consent. Just because she had given consent to some physical contact, she didn't know to take it back when she wanted it all to stop. Instead, Lauren froze. Far too many people use that lack of outright refusal as proof of consent, but that couldn't be further from the truth. Dr. Megan Maas, who teaches human sexuality at Michigan State University, broke it down for me. "You hear this all the time: Why didn't she say something? Why didn't she leave? Why didn't she punch him in the face?" she tells me. "And what a lot of people don't understand is that when you're in a traumatic situation, it's not just fight or flight. It's fight, flight, or freeze. And most women will report in sexual trauma that they'll freeze. It's a very natural response. I mean, other mammals do it when they're in a situation where they can't fight or flee. They'll freeze to play dead."

As grim as that sounds, it underscores an important point. It's not your fault if you couldn't say no when you wanted to. There are hundreds of factors, both personal and cultural, that implore women to be accommodating and nonconfrontational. Lauren mused to me that she was always taught to be a good hostess. But if you take one thing away from my story and hers, let it be this: No one has the right to

> **Your body is not a cocktail party, and you are not the hostess.**

make you feel like sex is inevitable or owed. Your body is not a cocktail party, and you are not the hostess.

Truly believing that is easier said than done, I know. But if you've ever struggled with expressing what your boundaries are, the good news is there are ways to practice.

Am I Into This? A Mental Checklist.

HAVE I SET BOUNDARIES?

First step: Figure out those boundaries. Before you consent to something, it helps to know whether you like it, or, if you've never done it before, whether you trust the person you're with enough to try it for the first time. And if you just don't know, one way to find out is to ask yourself some questions. I'd start with, "Do I feel safe?" The answer should always be yes, full stop. Then, "Do I feel listened to and supported?" Ditto, yes and yes. It's hard to imagine someone would be receptive to your wants and needs if they're not really listening.

AM I PRESENT?

Next: Clue in to your body and mind. Once you're doing [insert sex thing], keep asking questions like, "Do I feel any pain?" Sometimes a new position can be a little uncomfortable, but real pain is a signal to stop ASAP. You should also check in to see if you're physically turned on. Asking yourself, "Does my body feel warm and loose?" can help you find out. Then try, "Is my mind mostly relaxed?" This should be a yes, but it's okay to be a little nervous.

DO I REALLY WANT TO BE HERE?

If you feel a sense of relief at the thought of an "easy out" for this hookup, it's a good indicator this isn't the right time, place, or person for you. Like, "If the fire alarm went off and we had to leave this dorm right now, would I be relieved or bummed?" Finally, ask yourself "Am I performing?" and try to be honest.

"Am I performing?" is the one I'm most guilty of answering as no, when the answer was probably yes. Women are inundated with images of what it means to be "sexy" for their partner, whether it's Kylie Jenner's massive, pouty lips or the way a porn star arches her back mid–blow job. And so, as Dr. Maas points out, it's crucial to check in with yourself about whether you're doing something in bed to perform for someone else or because you really like how it feels. I think back to the cheap, acrylic lingerie I put on under my hoodie and sweats to surprise Jacob. It scratched and chafed and I felt kind of pathetic going through this song and dance for him, but I did it anyway because I'm sure I read somewhere that guys like that kind of thing.

⚠️ **All this to say: Don't let someone else's expectation of what's hot cloud your perception of what you actually like. If you think you're performing in bed, take a step back and ask yourself why.**

WITHDRAWING CONSENT

What to Do When It Stops Feeling Good

In a perfect world, every partner would be a master of consent. They would check in with you by whispering sexily in your ear, "Can I touch you there?" and you would feel totally confident indicating, "Hell yes, you can definitely touch me there." But the world isn't perfect. The reality is you'll probably sleep with people in your lifetime who haven't even heard of consent, let alone considered how to get better at giving and getting it. Even if you make your wishes totally clear, you may still have partners who outright ignore you and force themselves on you; that's sexual assault, without question, and we'll be discussing it in depth later on in this book.

But back to the million-dollar question. Everyone knows from a young age what to do when you suddenly catch on fire: Stop, drop, and roll. But what about when you find yourself in a sexual situation that's cooling off into no-longer-wanted territory?

If you didn't have a quick answer to that, you're not alone—and you're also not to blame. As a society, you'd think, we'd all be on board with the idea that you can stop being intimate with someone at any time, but nope! One recent UK-based survey[3] indicated that less than half of the respondents felt it was okay for someone to withdraw consent once they were naked. That number should be 100 percent. Another self-reported survey of 1,000 Americans showed that 1 out of every 8 women didn't believe she had the right to withdraw consent if she was already having sex. That means 1 out of every 8 of your friends has the mistaken notion that her body is not her own. Worse still, in North Carolina, it's currently illegal for a woman to withdraw consent once intercourse has begun. You read that right. So how are you supposed to feel confident responding to your body and changing your mind if the rest of the world is telling you that you can't? It's no small wonder that withdrawing consent is a lot more complicated than giving it. Many of my friends have told me they didn't withdraw consent during sex they really weren't into simply because they didn't want to ruin the possibility of a romantic future with their partner. But sex should never feel like a YouTube ad you're just waiting to finish. And while there's no tried-and-true method to turn your yes into a no, you've got a few options.

VERBALLY REDIRECT THEM

First you can try to verbally redirect your partner back to something that *did* feel good. That's why, according to Dr. Maas, it's so important to stay focused on positive sensations during sex—the contrast helps you become more aware of what isn't working. So let's say your partner has started fingering you in a penetrative way when they were just stroking your vulva moments before. You've consented to genital touching, but not like this. You don't want the hookup to end, but this is not good for you anymore. Help! Take a step back and focus on what felt good previously. Talk. You can try saying something like, "Hey, it was so hot the way you were touching me before, can we go back to that?"

Yes, that's hard to do, and for good reason. "One of the traps that a lot of women fall into is feeling like feedback equals direction," Vanessa Marin explains, which can be really intimidating if you feel pressure to explain to your partner exactly how to get you off. But you don't need to get that specific here. No one is expecting you to calmly proclaim, "Please, good sir, gently tap my clitoris in a counterclockwise circular motion while humming Cardi B's 'WAP'"! But redirecting with a quick sentence is a crucial strategy to practice. Ask yourself, "What did I like before?" and let your partner know.

SPEAK UP THROUGHOUT SEX

I firmly believe being able to talk about sex is the best possible way to make it better. In my experience, verbal consent is the most reliable strategy with a new hookup in particular. Moans and other nonverbal indicators of pleasure, as previously noted, are a great way to let someone know you like something, but with someone you've just met and who doesn't know your cues well, it's harder for them to pick up on the more subtle signs of consent. Marin explains that it's absolutely up to everyone to pay attention to the sounds and feelings someone is nonverbally giving off during sex—"I'm not a mind reader!" isn't an excuse for not paying attention at all—but nonverbal consent has its flaws. "I think it really works best when you're with a partner who you already know, trust, and have some sort of established connection with," she says. "Even a person who does know you might still misread what your signals are." That said, speaking up during sex is hard, and simply not possible for everyone at first, and you need strategies that will meet you where you are.

PHYSICALLY REDIRECT THEM

Dr. Liz Powell, a kink-friendly and sex-positive psychologist, recommends that if something stops feeling good or if your partner tries something you haven't consented to, you can physically redirect them. So let's go back to our Sad Sorry Fingering example. If you've decided you're done with your partner touching your vulva all together, you can grab their hand and move it up to your breasts, give it a squeeze, and make a sound to let them know, "Yes, please, much better."

If you're able to course correct by leading your partner back to a sexual act you like and consent to, great! But unfortunately, even when you've been crystal clear about your boundaries, it won't always work out that way. Whether your partner is just missing your signals or pressuring you to change your mind, sometimes the best thing you can do is to believe in your God-given right to leave them, naked and whining, in that bed.

WHEN ALL ELSE FAILS, GO TO THE BATHROOM

As much as women are socialized to feel guilt, male privilege entitles men to feel, well, entitled, to you and your body. They might complain of blue balls (not a real condition) or implore you to just stay a little longer: These are signs that your partner truly isn't hearing you. Society has a long way to go in fixing this, starting with men holding one another accountable for this misogynistic attitude. But you are *more* than entitled to leave any sexual situation that isn't fun for you. I can't pretend it will always be easy or even possible to do so. Sometimes you might feel too scared, or unsafe, or even frozen—that's awful, and it's not your fault. But when you can, try. If you need something to say, feel free to use, "Hey, I'm just not into this right now and I'm gonna head home."

If that's still too hard, Dr. Powell has another brilliant tip. Just say you need to go to the bathroom—or, if you're like me and the thought of someone considering you using the toilet fills you with anxiety, say you're going to get a drink of water. Why does this work so well? "If you need to go to the bathroom, no one's going to ask why," Powell explains. "It's the easiest way to escape from a situation that's not working." Once you're there, give yourself a breather so you can figure out your next steps. Maybe it involves bolting, maybe it'll give you a moment to decide how you're going to tell your partner you're leaving. No matter what you choose, taking yourself out of the heat of the moment gives you more space to think clearly. Bring your cellphone in there if you can. Call a friend and fake an emergency or a headache if that's what you need to do.

Even though Sabrina admits that she struggles to define consent, she's already used these tactics to her advantage when it comes to withdrawing it. She told me about a party she went to shortly before her first year of college. Her friend really wanted to hook up with a guy there, and his friend was interested in Sabrina, so she agreed to come along and play wingman. As the night wore on and the drinks added up, Sabrina and the guy who liked her wound up in one of the house's bedrooms. They were lying down, making out, feeling each other up, and all was more or less well. Sabrina explained he wasn't the hottest guy ever, but she was having a fun enough time. But then he tried to take off her pants, intimating that he wanted to have sex. By the time she had sobered up a bit and started telling him no, he kept pressing. "He definitely didn't just say okay when I didn't want to," she tells me. This is where men can intentionally muddy the waters of consent: by treating a "no" like an "ask again later." I call this "pulling a magic eight ball," and for the record, it's not okay.

Sabrina lied and said she was on her period, but still no dice. By this time, the idea of continuing to make out with him felt "gross," and she wanted to revoke consent for what she was originally fine with doing. Ultimately, he kept on pressuring her until she left the room and texted her friend that she wanted to leave. Sabrina's friend came down to meet her in the living room, where they made a swift exit. "We're never doing this again," Sabrina told her.

⚠️ **Getting yourself out of a bad situation is more important than what you had to say or do to make it possible. And if you can do it once or twice, you'll feel more confident about expressing your boundaries every other time.**

If Talking about Consent Is Still Hard for You, Your Friends Can Help

If your closest friends have carried out a full conversation in a bathroom stall over the sounds of you peeing, lent you their favorite bra, or cursed out every ex who ever broke your heart, they can help with this, too.

While it's true your parents and trusted adults are your first line of defense when it comes to talking about sex and consent, they don't always get those conversations right. Raise your hand if your sex talk with your mom consisted of her figuring out you'd already lost your virginity and then proceeding to awkwardly ignore you for a couple days! Just me?

If you're in my boat, friends can step in to offer support and accountability, too. We're all too quick to recount our sexual exploits with friends, but we don't always call them out if they've made a questionable hookup decision. Basically, when your face is broken out in zits and you got an awful haircut, your friends are the first to tell you to shut up because they know you're gorgeous. What if we provided that same kind of unconditional support and even tough love to one another when it comes to sex?

I have an incredible group of girlfriends who helped me survive college, and yes, we were always quick to come to the defense of a squad member who'd been romantically wronged. One time, a friend of mine even kicked a guy down a (small!) flight of stairs because he had been drunkenly flirting with two of us during the same night. (I don't advise that, by the way, but if you'd have been there, you'd have agreed it was awesome.) We practically went hoarse from all the times we screamed, "He doesn't deserve you!" through mascara-drenched tears. But what if we had pushed those conversations just a little deeper?

What if, over bagels in the dining hall, after one of our friends described a hookup that really wasn't good for her, we asked her why? What didn't she like about it? Especially for women who get uncomfortable telling a partner what they do and don't want in bed, reflecting on their feelings and practicing the act of saying it aloud to friends is a step to building more confidence when it comes to consent.

If your friend tells you she wasn't having a good time with a guy but spent the night anyway, gently ask her why she stayed. And if she says that she felt like she had already gotten that far so she might as well, or because she felt guilty, or because she didn't want to hurt his feelings, then you can tell her it doesn't have to be like that the next time. Just because she consented to make out with him doesn't mean she has to sleep with him. Sometimes it's easier to give your friends the advice you really need yourself, but if you hear it often enough, you can start believing it, too.

You can also help each other spot flags before they turn red. When you're out at a party and you see a guy innocently messing with, rough-housing with, or "playfully" tickling a girl and she's saying "Stop!" but he's not stopping, it might not be that innocent after all. Make a mental note. Let your friends know what you saw, because, as Vanessa Marin points out, that could be a sign of someone who doesn't take consent seriously, or at the very least "isn't clued in to the dynamics" around consent. She adds that these red flags can occur even over the phone. Say you're desperately trying to finish up the last few paragraphs of a paper before it's due and a guy you just met keeps texting you, even after you've said you're on a deadline. He just won't stop texting, and he seems annoyed you're not paying attention to him. That's another signal this is someone who might have trouble taking your requests seriously in a sexual context.

⚠️ **At the heart of these examples is someone who's prioritizing their own enjoyment over your boundaries. Get your friends to identify this behavior and get one another thinking about why it matters.**

But never stop telling one another that you're way too good for him, too.

ℓℓℓℓ

Maybe the reason I'll never forget where I was the first time a man blamed his erectile dysfunction on me isn't because of the absurdity or the cruelty of it. Maybe it was because it's the first time I can remember wishing in my head that my body was doing something other than what it was actually doing. It wasn't the last time, either. After freshman year ended and I moved off Jacob's floor, I pushed him out of my mind almost completely. He didn't enter my brain again until a year or two after I graduated.

I was living in Manhattan, out at a bar wearing shoes that hurt and was drinking cocktails I couldn't afford with my friends. After too many of said cocktails, I found myself in a cab with a guy I had been flirting with, and then in his bed. With the sounds of the city blaring through the open window, I heard him explain he didn't have a condom. There was no offer to run to the bodega and buy some, and no hint that we should slow things down, either. Somehow, I grabbed my clothes and blurted, "I have to go," to an extremely confused half-naked guy who maybe worked for Morgan Stanley? But who knows.

I didn't explain anything eloquently. I didn't use any of the tips you just read. I couldn't convey that if we didn't have protection, I wanted to remove myself from the situation before I felt pressured into doing something I'd regret. It was awkward and uncomfortable, but as I was searching for my shoes on this guy's floor, I remembered being in Jacob's bed. My insides burned as I flashed back to what it felt like to stay when you really wanted to go. With a mix of hesitancy and now, finally, a bit of rage, I realized I didn't owe this guy shit. I knew I wanted to be home more than anything else in the world at that moment, and I said what I could to get myself there.

It wasn't perfect, but it was progress.

2.

STIs

The "S" Doesn't Stand for "Shame"

"**C**an you just . . . can you just please look at my butt?" I asked my confused, skeptical boyfriend. Squinting in the fluorescent glow of my dimly lit dorm, he dutifully but hesitantly spread my butt cheeks to examine a few small red dots while the stars of *Sex and the City* smized at us from a poster above my bed. (Please be kind, it was 2009.)

I knew that before we got together, my then-boyfriend had an STI scare with another partner. (Just a heads-up here: STI is the acronym for "sexually transmitted infection." Some people still call them "sexually transmitted diseases," or STDs, but we'll talk about that later.)

This other young woman wound up testing positive for herpes, but all his panels were negative and he never had an outbreak. So when I saw the marks crop up months later, I panicked and wanted him to assess ASAP. Despite having little to no understanding of incubation periods for varying STIs, and despite his clear, repeated test results, and despite the fact that we'd never done anything butt-related sex-wise, I was in full-on hypochondriac paranoia.

When my then-boyfriend explained that he didn't think I had anything to worry about but that he, "uh, wasn't a doctor," we both decided to get retested. I fumed at him for days until the nurses at our college's student health center could see me. I had convinced myself that he had knowingly put my health at risk and alternated the silent treatment with sending him spiteful texts. "This is all your fault," I seethed.

I arrived at the on-campus clinic in tears and continued to dry heave my way through the blood test. The nurse on duty that day was mercifully patient with my hysterics, explaining to me that she understood how unsettling this was. "Herpes is a very emotional diagnosis," she said. Seven years out of college and that word still sticks with me: emotional. We both felt it: stress and despair from me, nervous anticipation and guilt from my boyfriend. We dragged all that heartache through the doors of that clinic, just as countless others did at colleges across the country, in part because we don't know how to talk about STIs without shame and judgment.

It turned out that the red marks were not herpes, but the result of ingrown hairs from a particularly far-reaching bikini wax. Whoops. I sheepishly apologized to my boyfriend about how worked up I'd gotten. Even though I take my sexual health seriously, he didn't deserve my vitriol. Then I stopped acknowledging it ever happened, just expecting he'd be able to forgive me. I had no idea just how clueless I'd been acting, but I would learn soon enough.

At that point in my life, all I had learned about STIs was that they were gross-looking and you should avoid people who have them at all costs, to protect yourself. This is a bad outlook for a lot of reasons, not least of all because it gives us fearful, negative attitudes about sex, but also because it makes us look at our peers who picked up an STI somewhere on their sex journey as dirty and irresponsible—I was definitely guilty of that. Not only did I torture my poor ex-boyfriend by being completely cruel when he was probably feeling just as nervous as I was, but I gossiped viciously about other people's sexual history when I was in college. When rumor broke about another girl who came down with herpes, I whispered to my friends in mock pity about how sad it was that her life was over. I was, for the record, an asshole, and I couldn't have been more wrong.

So perhaps it was karma that came for me late one night a few years after this incident. It was postcollege, and a couple of weeks prior, an ex of mine was in town and it seemed only appropriate that we reminisce with some halfhearted groping and a "you look well" blow job. He left the city and likewise my thoughts until an ill-fated night a couple weeks later when he called me up and melodramatically declared I needed to get tested. I freaked while I waited for him to say what for, fearing the worst. When he told me "chlamydia," I relaxed a bit.

Having learned from my Unjustified STI Meltdown in college, I did my best to keep calm. With my voice steady, I thanked him for letting me know and ended the call. But my faux chill dissipated quickly.

"Fuck," it dawned on me seconds later. "I might have to call Tom." Tom was a bit of an anomaly on my dating résumé at the time, and I was completely obsessed with him. Because I went to a liberal arts college, we didn't have football stars or "big men on campus." We didn't even have fraternities. I can't complain, I picked my alma mater for precisely the lack of Greek life, but the unintended result was that the theater guys and a cappella stars wound up filling the role of campus gods— often undeservedly so.

Tom was one of those guys. In college he had his pick of just about any girl within a five-mile radius of campus, and that never included me. Instead, I giddily watched him perform onstage, with my friends in the audience, chugging bottles of Diet Pepsi that were 60 percent cheap vodka. Never in my life did I think someone with that kind of confidence and magnetic charm would be interested in me. I was half right.

Tom and I never had so much as a conversation in college, but a year or two after graduating we met at a house party. I had stopped thinking about how cool he'd been and started believing how cool I had become postgrad (I had a job! I was on my way to becoming a writer! I had learned how to do a smoky eye from a YouTube tutorial!). I hit on him shamelessly in front of a large group of people in the living room of a cramped Manhattan apartment, and it actually worked.

That flirting led to a one-night stand, which may or may not have happened more than once. We were in that wonderful honeymoon stage of hooking up with a new partner, where everything is calculated texts full of heightened anticipation and blissful "holy shit I didn't know my body could bend that way" sex revelations, when I had to deliver the news.

I had gone to my doctor thinking it was unlikely I'd be positive for chlamydia. After all, I'd only had oral sex with my ex, and I assumed the risk was much lower. For an entire week at work, the thought hovered just out of frame as my mind faded in and out with what-ifs. But after several days, my results were finally ready. On my way home from the office, I stood in a crowded, noisy subway station, getting pushed around by restless New Yorkers. Suddenly, my phone lit up with my doctor's number. "It seems you were positive for . . . what we were discussing the other day," she said to me quietly.

Was it so bad she couldn't even say the word out loud? I wondered. I pressed my cell closer to my ear, struggling to find a private nook of the subway station to talk about my newly infected private nook. I felt a rolling wave of nausea shoot up from my stomach and linger in my throat as I listened to my doctor explain when my prescription would be ready and how to take it. After squeaking out a "thanks," we hung up.

A little shell-shocked, I bumped through the crowds of people on the train without even registering their scowls and went directly to my pharmacy. With two out of three unpleasant phone calls done, I knew there was one more.

Sitting with my legs crossed on my bed and completely petrified, I texted Tom, who I had seen a week ago. "Hey, do you have a minute?"—a very casual line that I agonized over for at least twelve minutes, meant to convey a certain amount of chill but still telegraph the gravitas of the call I was about to make.

He told me he was out to dinner with a friend (What luck! Another hot guy I went to college with can be present to joke about what a slut I am!) and that he needed to make it quick. So I got right to the point, told him he needed to get tested, and reiterated how easy the treatment was with antibiotics. The exchange was brief, though I recall his being kind in a slightly underhanded way. "This stuff is just par for the course for people like us, you know? Don't worry about it, I know the drill," he told me with a nonchalance that was both comforting and off-putting.

And even though the subtext was "hahaha, us sexually active, dirty whores can't be bothered by mere infections!," it registered with a pang of regret that he was still eons nicer than I had been to my ex in college.

The remark stung for so many reasons. Every ignorant "better her than me" line I uttered about people I knew with STIs came hurling back in my direction, sent from my own hand. With what I thought was the worst of the night behind me, I swallowed my antibiotics and cried with relief and pent-up stress. But the worst was not over. Antibiotics don't fix *everything*. I was wrong about that, and unfortunately, so many other young adults are, too.

HOW DID WE GET SO SCARED OF STIs?

Let's start with your high school sex ed: It probably sucked. I'm hard on myself for how obtuse I was about STIs in college, but at that point in my life, why wouldn't I have panicked? Although one out of every five[1] Americans has an STI, and half of the new yearly cases are people ages fifteen to twenty-four, the stigma surrounding them is palpable. And it starts young. High school sex ed traumatized me, and undoubtedly my peers, with images of swollen, mangled genitalia presented as the nasty, unavoidable consequence of sex. I sat in class in horror as a teacher explained to me there were some diseases that never, ever went away. She unpacked how if you got one, you'd have to explain your "condition" to every sexual partner you had for the rest of your life. Sure, this is true in some instances, but it was always the most extreme cases that made it to the lesson plan. There was not one mention of managing an STI with medication, or how people with chronic STIs still lead productive, happy, partnered lives (duh). And now seems like a pretty good time to reiterate: I grew up in progressive New England. I had comparatively good sex ed. Like, abstinence-is-unrealistic, here's-how-to-put-a-condom-on-a-banana good. And still I was left with the impression that anyone with an STI was some dirty, social pariah.

I hear stories of the schooling my friends received in other parts of the country and it's really no wonder at all how we wound up this way. My friend Emily shared how she distinctly recalls her health teacher telling her that you could physically feel your ovaries release an egg during ovulation "if you sat still." Which, no. Another friend, Alex, shared some of my visual trauma, citing a textbook with "a picture of a penis that honest to god looked like it had cauliflower growing out of it." Then there's Serena, who graduated in 2018 from Texas State University and got her "sex ed" from her Catholic high school. In a lesson plan titled Operation Keepsake—yes, as in "your virginity is a keepsake that should remain sequestered in a glass display cabinet"—she recalls the teachers placing a Hershey's Kiss on every student's desk. Then, teachers told the class: "You are not allowed to touch this. This is the temptation of sex. You really want to touch it, but you are not allowed to until you're married." She told me this lesson was "the dumbest thing" she'd ever heard, but the problem runs much deeper than just an ignorant metaphor. "There was no talk of condoms or things like that," Serena explained. "STDs were like a sin in Catholic school. We never talked about that."

And even though my sex ed was some fifteen years ago, what still goes on in classrooms today is shocking. While some states have banned abstinence-only sex ed, many still preach extremely sex-negative and harmful gospel. Some lessons[2] in use now involve asking students to choose a fresh piece of candy from a bag, suck on it, then rewrap it and put it back in the bag. Then that same bag is presented to another student, forcing them to choose: Do you want a "used" candy or a "fresh" candy? The implication that having sex makes you "used up" is problematic enough on its own. Then there are the still-currently-taught[3] lesson plans that showcase a dejected woman bemoaning how one case of gonorrhea left her barren and childless for life, all because her future husband didn't wait until marriage. In truth, this side effect is very rare. Yes, gonorrhea and chlamydia can lead to pelvic inflammatory disease and infertility *if left untreated*, but even then, that only occurs in 10 to 15 percent[4] of untreated cases of chlamydia. While such lessons may be taught in the guise of explaining disease transmission, it sends a pretty clear message that having sex (and God forbid, getting an infection) is somehow dirty.

So why, when so many STIs are easily curable, do we use the example of the woman who became infertile after her chlamydia diagnosis, instead of one like mine? Well, to scare you into caring about protection. To put it simply, if you can avoid getting an STI, you should. But in using a model of risk reduction, sexuality researcher Dr. Shayna

Skakoon-Sparling, PhD, notes, we often completely sidestep giving practical education. "When you're telling people 'don't have sex,' they aren't planning for sex. And when you weren't planning for sex, you don't have any condoms with you, because you were trying to follow the adults' instructions who told you 'just don't have sex.'" Shocking to no one: If you don't use condoms, your likelihood of getting an STI is much higher. Dr. Sparling uses a metaphor I love for abstinence-centered, fear-based sex ed. She says it's like telling people not to cook in their kitchen. If they don't know how to use a stove, when they inevitably get hungry and turn it on, they're going to get burned.

It's possible some of the educators who create these scary sex ed curricula have their hearts in the right place. Gynecologist and author Dr. Alyssa Dweck notes that anti-smoking ad campaigns that used graphic images of the harmful outcomes of cigarettes were effective,[5] and posits that perhaps some of that logic has been applied to what we teach young adults about sex. But, she explains, "this kind of scary, 'tough love' approach could be stigmatizing and traumatic given the sensitive subject matter, especially for anyone who has had an STI." After all, you can live a perfectly happy, healthy life without cigarettes. You can't necessarily say the same about sex.

What's more, scary photos of the advanced stages of a herpes outbreak, for example, might not only frighten students and intimidate them out of getting tested, but it can also lead to a damaging, false sense of confidence when it comes to identifying STIs. "By showing kids those images, we're also screwing people over in another way because they think that now they're always going to be able to tell. Like, 'Oh, I had sex with that guy last weekend, his genitals looked totally fine,'" Dr. Sparling explains. Thinking every STI is going to look like the photos you saw in health class could lead you to believe that you can physically determine with the naked eye who has an STI and who does not. That couldn't be further from the truth. Lots of STIs, like gonorrhea and chlamydia, can have no symptoms at all.

Let's also not pretend infections like herpes haven't been the butt of the joke for ages. Even progressive, forward-thinking comedies with women at the helm like *Parks and Recreation* use herpes as a punchline now and then. When everyone around you treats STIs like a sad, scary, funny, undesirable condition, why wouldn't you?

STIs 101

The Bare-Minimum Basics

You could fill entire textbooks with the symptoms, treatments, and incubation periods for every single sexually transmitted infection in the known universe. For better or worse, this is not that book. What I can offer you here are four basic concepts that will help you take control of your sexual health.

1. Get tested, often.

Seriously! It's one of the most important things you can do to keep yourself healthy. Dr. Leah Millheiser, director of the Female Sexual Medicine Program at Stanford University Medical Center, recommends that all sexually active people be tested for gonorrhea and chlamydia yearly, prior to the age of twenty-five, when they're at the highest risk for those infections. From ages twenty-one to twenty-nine, women should get a pap smear every three years to screen for human papillomavirus (HPV) and signs of cervical cancer. If you've never had a pap smear, while not exactly thrilling, it falls somewhere around "slightly uncomfortable" on the spectrum of doctor experiences. Your gynecologist will insert a device called a speculum that opens the walls of your vagina, and then collect a cell sample from your cervix. It feels like a light scraping sensation and is over super quickly. (I am someone who routinely anxiety-faints at the doctor's office, but I get through these with no problem, so I promise you can, too.)

Dr. Millheiser explains that in a perfect world, you'd get tested before every new sexual partner. Great in theory, but in my wildest of nights, I'm not embarrassed to say (though not exactly proud, either) that I had sex with more than one person in a 24-hour period. There literally wouldn't have been enough time to get to the clinic, let alone for the results to come through. It's not a secret that the hookup scene drives most relationships in college, and hookups can be thrilling, unexpected, and impulsive. But they can also be unsafe if you don't know your STI status. So Dr. Sparling has a suggestion you probably didn't hear in your health class: If you're having sex with multiple partners on the regular, just get tested at least every three months as a general guide. That way, if you do pick up an STI, especially one without symptoms, you'll find out relatively quickly and avoid complications. Be sure to ask for a full panel of STI testing so you can be certain you're checking for STIs like syphilis as well, which is currently on the rise.[6]

2. Use condoms.

Okay, this one you probably *have* heard in health class before. But it's still important. A condom is called a "barrier method" for good reason: It provides a barrier between you and STIs (and unwanted pregnancy). And yes, if you're monogamous with a partner and you've both shared your STI status, you can certainly discuss ceasing condom use—provided you have backup birth control like the pill or an IUD. But even in the most trusting of relationships, STIs can still occur. For example, according to Dr. Millheiser, herpes likely won't show up in someone's blood work for a month after exposure, so the results you're seeing might not be totally accurate, depending on when they were tested. And as much as it might hurt to acknowledge, people lie. Especially—and this is only in my experience, don't push me for hard data here—college-age men who are about to put their penis inside someone. Dr. Millheiser has seen this all too often. "[There's] that small chance that maybe your partner wasn't faithful. . . . I have seen many college-age women who have gotten STDs because they were told by their partner, 'Oh no, no, no, I had a clean bill of health a couple months ago. We're good.' And they come in with an STD. So, don't take someone's word at face value." When the sex is casual, use a condom. Period.

3. STIs are complicated.

Here's a fun paradox: While there's way too much puritanical panic around STIs, the truth is that getting any kind of infection isn't a "desirable outcome," as Dr. Sparling puts it. Because of the possibility of complications, protection and testing are your first line of defense. Not to sound like an after-school special, but gonorrhea and chlamydia, for example, *can* lead to pelvic inflammatory disease and even infertility. While that's not common, the point is that it can still happen. And because both of those infections can have no symptoms at all in women, you may not ever know you have it if you're not getting tested regularly. That's why you hear about the scary examples. It's not that there's anything wrong with sex; it's that those risks *are* possible. Beyond being intellectually and physically complicated, STIs can often act in ways you might not expect. While less common, a small cold sore on someone's mouth can be transmitted and become genital herpes on their partner if they're having oral sex. And I am a walking, talking billboard against assuming something is safer than it is. I figured the risk of infection in unprotected oral sex would be almost impossible, but I still got chlamydia after giving an ex a blow job. If nothing else, let that be a reminder that sex with your ex is almost never worth it.

4. Your sex life isn't over if you get an STI.

Really! Even a chronic infection. If you get diagnosed with an STI like gonorrhea or chlamydia, you can treat it easily with a prescription, and you'll never be obligated to disclose that to a partner again. Or, if you're like me, you can put it in a book. Your choice. But even herpes, which I feared and misunderstood in equal parts in college, isn't the death sentence I thought it was. Suppressive medications like Valtrex can reduce the number of breakouts you have and decrease "viral shedding," the process through which infection transmits to a partner, even when you're asymptomatic. Taking such meds can greatly lower[7] your risk of transmission. Yes, having to tell future partners about your diagnosis does add an extra layer of communication that could potentially complicate things, but it's so much less of a big deal than your sex ed teacher probably made it out to be.

Joanna, now twenty-six, found out she got herpes right before her junior year of college at a liberal arts school in the Northeast. "I woke up on Thursday morning, and something was not right. I was in a lot of pain, and when I poked around down there, I saw a bunch of raised red and white sores that were painful to touch. So like any freaked-out millennial, I went straight to Google and tried to figure out what my symptoms might be. And pretty conclusively, Google was like, you probably have genital herpes. So I called my student health clinic and set up an appointment for that afternoon." In the hours between, Joanna was panicking. "I'm not a religious person, but I was definitely doing that kind of bargaining where it's like, 'If this isn't genital herpes, I promise I will actually study for my exam.'" But after the nurses at her student health center did a swab of a lesion, she knew for sure that it was. Not every sexual partner will react kindly to this kind of news, and her boyfriend at the time certainly didn't. Because Joanna had had more sexual partners than he did, he immediately began lashing out, even telling her,

"This is what I get for falling for a girl like you." As painful as it was, she didn't let it break her down. This isn't to say Joanna didn't have to do some work coming to terms with suddenly feeling alien in her own body. But by steeling up her confidence and embracing a strategy of blurting out her diagnosis in a casual way, by Halloween, she was back out at parties and hooking up with people, just as junior year might typically be. Since then, she's found that if she's just direct, people are so much more chill about it than she thought they'd be. After all, more than one out of every six people has herpes.[8] Chances are you have friends and family who have it, too.

And hey, if you get an STI and need some time to process it, there's no rule that says you have to immediately get back out there, either. Take Dawn, twenty-two, who just graduated from Arizona State University. Dawn was just becoming sexually active her sophomore year when she contracted herpes from a guy she knew through work. What's worse, it eventually became clear to Dawn that he knew his status prior to their hookup and didn't tell her. (Take note: Willfully refusing to disclose is a crime, so . . . don't do that.) When she noticed her symptoms, she booked the first online appointment she could at her local clinic. Unlike Joanna, who had a relatively positive experience with the doctor who diagnosed her, Dawn's doctor spoke to her in a pitying and condescending tone. She says he broke the news in "the saddest voice ever. It was like, *Shit, that doesn't feel so great*," Dawn recalls. Since then, Dawn says the hardest part of her journey has been dealing with the stigma. It wears on her when she hears herpes mentioned as the worst-case scenario punchline in a rom com, or when she overhears people calling cold sores gross. The whole situation brought up anxiety and feelings of inadequacy that she'd been struggling with her whole life, but she didn't crumble under the weight of it. Dawn ditched the clinic creep of a doctor, found herself a sex-positive gynecologist, and got into therapy to deal with her feelings. "It doesn't affect my life in any other way. The stigma isn't really as strong when you're talking to someone one on one, and they see you as a person. I've told friends and my family and they're so sweet and kind and not judgmental about it. I'm not treated differently because of it." Dawn isn't ready to start having sex again, but she has the support system in place to help her feel empowered to have the conversations she'll need to when she does.

STIs 201

How to Have the Tricky Conversations

So, STIs are super common, and you'll probably get one, but no one prepares you for how to talk about them. The two most common STI conversations you'll need to have are asking someone about their status, and alerting them of yours. Here's how.

ASKING ABOUT THEIR STATUS

If you're about to have sex with a new partner, do your best to have the STI talk before your clothes come off. This is simply because it's easier to think straight when you're not naked! It takes the pressure off both of you to make serious decisions in the heat of the moment. Joanna has some practical advice for wording, too. She likes to ask, "Do you know your STI status?" to kick off the conversation. Asking someone, "When was the last time you were tested?" can feel a bit more aggressive and almost like a pop quiz. Opening the conversation in a more neutral way is a good start to honest disclosure.

Remember that it's your right, and even an obligation to yourself, to ask that question. Dr. Millheiser explains that all too often, young women in particular don't feel empowered to ask the questions that help them protect their sexual health. Maybe, she notes, they're worried about scaring a partner away by putting up barriers to a sexual relationship. Or maybe just by asking about testing, it implies that they've slept around. This is just another way rigid, regressive opinions about sexually active young women actually put us at risk. So consider carefully how your partner reacts to your query. Any partner who gets scared away by your asking a simple question that you're one hundred percent entitled to ask probably has something to hide, even if it's just a misogynistic attitude.

DISCLOSING YOUR STATUS

All the experts I spoke to agreed on one point: If you need to tell someone else about your STI status, try and stay relaxed. Because, they explain, if you're crying and freaking out, you're likely going to put your partner in an emotionally charged state. This is basically a "monkey see, monkey do" scenario, wherein if you can stay calm and project the idea that this isn't a big deal, they'll be more likely to relax enough to hear what you're saying.

Another expert-approved tip is to be knowledgeable about your condition. So if you can say, for example, "I have genital herpes, I'm taking a suppressive medication, the risk of transmitting it to you is really low, and we can use condoms, too," that will assure your partner that you both take it seriously and have the situation handled responsibly. With herpes in particular, you'll likely learn the triggers that bring about an outbreak, like stress and even certain foods. That's just another way to better understand the condition and know which times are safer to have sex, and when you should avoid it.

But there's no denying these conversations are hard. If you find out you contracted an STI and need to retroactively tell a partner but just can't manage a phone call, there are even websites like stdcheck.com that will anonymously alert someone via text that they should get tested. Jenelle Marie Pierce founded and runs The STI Project, a multifaceted online resource that connects individuals who are STI-positive with a wealth of information about testing and firsthand stories about living with and talking about STIs. She's also an advocate for having these conversations over text message if that's what works best for you. More often than not, Pierce explains, people with STIs feel pressure to worry about and protect the sexual and emotional well-being of others, but they should be equally concerned about protecting themselves. Statistically, if you already have one STI, you're more likely to contract another, so if a potential partner seems too lax about condom use, that should be a red flag for you. "Your body is just as important, even with that STI," she says. And that's where texting comes in. Pierce explains that sometimes an in-person conversation about STI disclosure can put people on the spot, and they may make a decision they wouldn't have if they had some time to think about it. Plus, she says, having the conversation over text can spare you the momentary pain of someone who may have a negative reaction or make a weird facial expression if you disclose that you're positive for a certain STI. Your feelings matter here, too, and you deserve to have barriers that may help you protect your mental health.

If you're on the flip side of this and someone comes to you and responsibly discloses that they have an STI, be kind. They might be feeling scared, anxious, and overwhelmed. Talking about STIs can make us feel really vulnerable, so reacting with compassion is the least we can do for one another.

STIs 301

Beyond the Basics: How Can We Stop Feeling So Ashamed of STIs?

We need inclusive sex ed that gives practical advice and explains the treatment and management of STIs with honesty, and without the scare tactics. But until we get it, there's a lot you can do on your own. Having an STI, even though they're so incredibly common, can really make you feel alone. But the way we think and talk to one another about them can slowly change that. Think for just a moment on the difference between the term "sexually transmitted infection" and "sexually transmitted disease." The former feels temporary, less severe, not a threat to the people around you. The latter implies permanence and a heightened safety risk to others. Dr. Dweck notes that it's similar to the transition in how we talk about erectile dysfunction. Years ago we used to call it impotence, implying anyone who suffers from it is weak and has no power. Call it "ED," and it's not about you at all, it's about a part of you that's temporarily not working as it should.

Another verbal trap you can easily escape is saying you had a "clean" STI test when you really mean "negative." Someone who has an STI isn't dirty. The only determining factor that makes someone dirty is whether or not they've showered recently.

Dr. Sparling suggests that getting tested regularly is not only good for your health but great for shutting down STI stigma. If more people go through the process regularly, it won't seem so daunting for others. I avoided getting a blood test for HIV for six years after becoming sexually active because I was so afraid of the process and even more terrified of the answer. Had I gone earlier, I might have learned about drugs like PrEP, or pre-exposure prophylaxis, which, when taken every day, make it virtually impossible to contract HIV. Or even PEP, post-exposure prophylaxis, which when taken after potential exposure to HIV can prevent the virus from taking hold. Now that we know more, and the U = U (undetectable = untransmittable) campaign has become more visible, stigma may start to wane more and more. These advancements are especially crucial for the LGBTQ and Black communities, who are disproportionately affected by HIV.[9] In the past, when the stigma was especially high, people in these minority groups were unfairly looked at as vectors of disease and discriminated against in the workplace. Today, they may still be uncomfortable sharing their status or seeking testing due to judgmental treatment from healthcare providers, among other concerns. But these medical advancements give many a lot of hope. There's much to learn that can give you peace of mind if you're not too busy running from the facts.

Someone who credits being alive today to the advancements of HIV medication is Ashley, a twenty-three-year-old recent graduate who went to school in Toronto, Canada. Ashley was born with HIV and started her lifesaving medication before she truly understood her condition. Today she's a vocal advocate for HIV awareness and isn't shy about discussing her status, but even so, she has still experienced varying forms of stigma. Once, when she was visiting a mall while traveling to give a talk as a part of her advocacy work, her chatty mother mentioned the purpose of her trip to a cashier, who turned to then-sixteen-year-old Ashley and asked, "Are you okay?" She remembers thinking how weird it was that this stranger assumed she was frail and unwell just because she's HIV-positive, especially since she felt strong enough to travel the country and work. Beyond that, she explains, there's still this image of people with HIV as dirty or gross. Even more complicated is that there are varying layers of stigma depending on people's perceptions of how you contracted the virus. Those who contracted it through sex, rather than through birth, might experience more blame for what's perceived as their own "risky choices." This is crap, in case the quotes weren't clear, and Ashley agrees. "At the end of the day, HIV is HIV no matter how you get it. And you shouldn't be ashamed about how you did. Before my birth mom passed away, I was told that she had contracted it from unprotected sex from a man she thought she could trust. Hearing that as a kid, I didn't really understand it. But being a grown adult, I'm like, 'How could anyone shame someone for doing something so natural?'"

What could be more natural than love, intimacy, and wanting to believe our partners have our best interests at heart? Nowadays, Ashley doesn't think too much about her HIV status unless she's at a doctor's appointment or talking to someone about it. But when she does discuss it, with a romantic partner or otherwise, she recommends being direct and calm about it. In fact, she told her current boyfriend about her status the first night they met. They were out with a group of friends at McDonald's after a basketball game, and she cracked a joke about HIV (she doesn't recall exactly what it was). Her friends who knew her well laughed, but he looked a little confused. She told him what the deal was, and they spent the rest of the night eating french fries, joking, and laughing together. He asked her some questions, did his own research, and now even educates some of his friends about HIV. This is pretty much the ideal way to react to a partner's disclosure, she says. Ashley explains that she's a bit more cautious than the average person her age when it comes to protection and vetting partners—she likes to tell them early on, before anything trends too romantic, so she can test the waters of their reaction—but overall, HIV hasn't been some massive stumbling block in her relationships. With her medication, the levels of the virus in her body are so low she can't transmit it to anyone. She can have kids without passing it on to them, too. More education about the advances in medicine could really change the misconceptions we have about HIV, she suggests, but for now, she wants others living with it to feel confident sharing this piece of their identity with others: "Do whatever your heart's telling you but make sure you're comfortable and abiding by your own personal judgment, not judgments of other people."

All this to say, if you do develop an STI, especially in your college years, repeat this mantra: My sex life isn't over. Jenelle Marie Pierce has noticed, in her career, interviewing tons of young adults who are STI-positive for her website, that one of the biggest myths she encounters is that college students feel like these four years are the only chance to truly experiment and get to know yourself sexually. "There's this idea that as soon as you get the diagnosis, that gets stripped away," Pierce says. That couldn't be further from the truth for a number of reasons. For one, as you'll read later in this book, not everyone in college is out there having heaps of casual sex with a rotating cast of characters. For another, you can learn plenty about your sexual likes and dislikes from masturbation, or by trying new things with just one or two partners. And lastly, people with STIs who understand the risks and take steps to protect themselves go on to have tons of casual sex, if that's what they want. Your sex life isn't over, period.

Finally, don't talk shit about other people if you've heard that they have an STI. It sounds so simple, but in social situations it can be really hard to be the only one standing up against gossip, or saying you don't find a joke about herpes funny. The way we discuss STIs has the ability to affect people's lives, for better or worse. Let's make it better.

> **If you do develop an STI, repeat this mantra: My sex life isn't over.**

eeee

The night I took my antibiotics, I was living in an apartment with my mom and sister. What I wasn't prepared for is that the high dose of azithromycin required to kill a chlamydia infection can cause a seriously painful stomachache. Not knowing how bad it would be, in the minutes after I swallowed the pills with a glass of cranberry juice, I thought I'd be putting this whole thing behind me. But a couple of hours later I was curled up in a ball on my bed, clutching my knees to my chest in unbearable pain, trying not to let my family hear me crying. I was ten feet from the people who love me most in the world, and I still felt too alone, ashamed, and scared to tell them I was hurting.

After that moment, I knew I'd do everything I could to make sure no one I knew felt that way again. It was too late to take back the insults I yelled at my ex or the snarky jabs I'd made at other people's expense, but I could make a choice to handle things differently from here on out. I was a clueless bitch once. I didn't have to stay that way.

So now when I'm hanging out with my guy friends, I'm the stick-in-the-mud who asks them to "explain the funny part" about that stand-up special they love that makes fun of people with the clap. Now, when my group chat lights up with one of my girlfriends asking if anyone's ever had a colposcopy (basically a slightly more invasive pap smear to get a closer look if something seems abnormal), I answer. I'm the first to say yep, I've had one, this is what it's like, and you'll be totally fine.

3.

Cocktail Conundrums

When Liquid Courage Creates Sticky Situations

There is really no way to say this without sounding like some sort of bizarre humble-brag, but I never had any major problems with drinking when I was in college: I never blacked out, I threw up just once in four years of school, and I felt comfortable at parties even if I wasn't tipsy. I attribute this to a few factors. For one, all of my high school health classes had convinced me that if I got too wasted, I would die passed out on my back, choking on my vomit, full stop. On top of that, I once snuck a water bottle full of vodka that I stole from my parents' liquor cabinet (Sorry, Mom and Dad) into a sleepover with friends, with disastrous results. I was fine, but one girl spent the entire night puking, and even though lots of us had pilfered booze, I was convinced I had poisoned her and that she would die, and it would be all my fault. As a result, I developed what I considered to be a healthy fear of alcohol that prevented me from overdoing it most of the time. Again, it's not like I deserve a gold star, but given the horror stories I've heard—from waking up in puke-soaked party dresses to much worse—I feel lucky.

But that doesn't mean that the way I drank didn't present unanticipated complications when it came to sex. Drinking makes your brain fuzzier and can cause you to forget things. Important things. Things like, oh say, taking your birth control pill every night during roughly the same time window. (Which is a thing that happened to me not infrequently, in case you couldn't tell from my cagey, embarrassed tone.) And no, missing just one pill does not automatically result in an unplanned pregnancy, but repeated misuse of any contraceptive decreases its effectiveness, and that's really not a chance you want to take. Then there were the multiple occasions I woke up in someone else's dorm room with a burning sensation radiating from my vagina, like some sort of crotch-specific migraine. Why? Well, another side effect of drinking is feeling sleepy, which I felt after a night of booze and hooking up. I'd pass out, forget to pee after intercourse—which is widely believed[1] to help reduce your chance of a urinary tract infection—and wake up with the beginnings of an unbearable UTI. One night it was so awful that I woke up in pain at 5 AM, couldn't get back to sleep, and had to skip class in order to see a nurse right when our health center opened the next day. (This didn't sit well with me: I had done the math of how much each class cost and quickly realized I didn't want to be skipping them unless absolutely necessary.) Still, the stakes for me were not incredibly high: I was mostly responsible with my birth control, and I had easy access to antibiotics—but they were both unnecessary risks I wouldn't have taken if I were sober.

Beyond the privacy of your bedroom, drinking too much can complicate your social life, too. Nearly twelve years after the fact, I still remember a friend of a friend who met up with my gang of girls for Halloween one year. As we pregamed in our dorm room, she slowly became more and more drunk. Suddenly, she was enthusiastically making out with a guy who had come dressed as a clown wearing a full greasepaint-makeup getup. I will never object to public smooching at a party, but the problem was the aftermath. She was too drunk to notice his makeup had transferred all over her face, and she walked around for a not-insignificant amount of time with a thick black mustache of paint above her lip. After a laugh, we eventually got her cleaned up and taken care of, but even then I worried what would have happened if she hadn't been among friends. At a bigger party with less empathetic guests, people might not have told her, might have posted mocking photos, and what was a silly gaffe could have easily been a semitraumatic evening for someone who wasn't aware enough to take care of herself.

When it feels like drinking is college's national pastime, but you know there are risks involved, how do you take part while still protecting yourself, especially when sex is involved?

PARTYING 101
The Risks of College Drinking

Of course I don't advocate breaking the law and underage drinking, but I have been to college. I've done it. I've seen it. I'd venture to say it's happening nearly every night of the week on just about every campus in America. Just like withholding sex ed doesn't result in fewer unwanted pregnancies, we can't pretend teens aren't drinking if we want them to understand how to do it more safely. With that said, not to freak you out with scary numbers, but I'm going to freak you out with scary numbers. Alcohol is a huge part of sexual assault risk. Studies show that about half of college sexual assaults involve alcohol.[2] Some data suggests that up to 74 percent of perpetrators and 55 percent of victims were drinking when the assault happened. On top of that, when looking at assaults where alcohol was involved, both parties were drinking 97 percent of the time. This is obviously not to say that alcohol is the cause of sexual assault. You'll hear me say this more than once: The only thing all assaults have in common is someone who decided to assault another person. So yes, drinking isn't the cause, but it's a big contributing factor, and we'd be reckless to ignore it. I like to think about it this way: We all know even if you're the best, safest driver in the world, you could be in a car accident any time you get on the road. We just can't predict what other drivers will do, or what surprising conditions will take our safety out of our control. And just because you got into an accident doesn't necessarily make it your fault. However, being a responsible driver doesn't mean you wouldn't wear a seatbelt. Look, it's not a perfect metaphor, because assault is never a survivor's fault, but safe-drinking practices are like seatbelts when it comes to drinking and sex. You need to use them, because they help.

Sexual assault isn't the only risk factor of drinking too much. I spoke with Megan Patrick, PhD, a researcher studying alcohol and sexual health behaviors at the University of Michigan, who explains that another common, concerning problem when it comes to sex and drinking too much is waking up the next morning and not remembering what happened. While it might *seem* sexy to get to tell your friends, "Oh my god, I have no idea what Chad from the lacrosse team and I did last night!," it's actually super dangerous. If you can't remember what you did, you might not have asked your partner about STIs, used protection, or let your partner know if something they did hurt you. Rough sex—especially when sensation is physically dulled by alcohol and you can't accurately gauge force and pressure—can be dangerous. In general, if you ever wake up and can't remember everything but suspect or know sexual contact occurred the night before, get tested for STIs, and consider taking Plan B. An obvious exception to this rule is if you're on the pill or have an IUD, *and* your partner was someone whose STI status you know for a fact.

Margot, a junior at a large school in New York, knows how scary this can be firsthand. One night, she and a friend were at a bar when an older man approached them. Clearly uninterested in his advances, Margot and her friend were uncomfortable, at which point a couple of younger guys stepped in to intervene. Grateful for the assist, she remembers talking with them and taking shots, and then nothing else. The next day, she woke up in bed with one of the guys, and her friend was with the other on a futon on the floor. The pair of guys left around 7 AM, but Margot was shaken up. She wasn't certain whether or not they had sex, but her vagina was sore the next day. Margot didn't think this would have happened if she hadn't been so drunk. "I would have said no," she tells me. Trying to put it behind her, she didn't take Plan B or visit a doctor at the time, but told me after having had time to reflect, she absolutely would if something like this ever happened again. Things went from bad to worse when, a few weeks later, her dad was visiting her at school and accidentally discovered two vials of an illegal white drug in her futon. Putting together the pieces, Margot knew the only people who could have left them there were the guys who had come over that night. Since she blacked out, she had no way of knowing if they had taken any of those drugs together. The dangers are not always the obvious ones. You often have more to lose than you may think in the moment— say, a scholarship or your driver's license, if you're caught in the wrong situation. Thankfully she was able to work things out with her father, but had someone from her university found those drugs instead, the situation could have been far worse.

I'm grateful everything turned out okay for Margot and that she shared this vulnerable moment. After all, none of us "knows" any "better" until we've lived an experience and realized, "Wow. I could have handled that differently." The "knowing" comes from living, doing, talking, and thinking critically about how you can handle these situations. But Margot's story does illustrate a number of risks associated with drinking

> # The "knowing" comes from living, doing, talking, and thinking critically about how you can handle these situations.

and sex. For example, Megan Patrick explains that drinking can lead to not using a condom, or using a condom improperly. She also notes, as Margot felt, that drinking and sex can lead to a feeling that things moved faster than you wanted them to. This is not to say you should be ashamed of having casual sex—you shouldn't!—just that you should be able to dictate the sex you have and when you have it on your own terms, and drinking can drive you to make decisions you might not have made otherwise.

OKAY, SO WHY ARE WE STILL DOING THIS?

A lot of college students drink, regardless of who threw scary numbers and stories at them. (Guilty as charged!) But knowing the risks is a crucial bit of information that can help you decide what you want. So why is alcohol still so prevalent on college campuses? Turns out, the answer isn't super straightforward.

When you arrive on campus as a freshman and make it to your first weekend, it's easy to think that lit-er-al-ly everyone drinks. Party culture is loud, boisterous, and public. But the numbers tell a different story. According to data collected from campuses across the country in the Spring 2019 National College Health Assessment, about 56 percent of college students drank in the month prior to taking the survey.[3] That's a lot, even a slight majority, but it's certainly not everyone. And here's where a potential factor for why we drink so much comes into play. When asked, college students reported that they believed about 93 percent of their peers were drinking during the past 30 days, far higher than the actual 56 percent. Patrick explains that students' drinking habits may be trying to match their overestimation of their peers' drinking habits. So it's not just that students have inaccurate beliefs about what their friends are up to, it's that the inaccurate beliefs are causing them to drink a ton more to catch up to a lie. Repeat after me: No one is drinking as much as you think they are.

Then of course there's the idea that drinking will lead to fun or sex, often referred to as alcohol expectancy theory. According to Patrick, the idea is that whatever you believe alcohol will do for you will often have a self-fulfilling-prophecy effect—not because alcohol really does those things, but because you believe it does. So if there's a group of people all in one concentrated area who think booze, rather than friends, music, conversation, snacks, and dancing are what make a party fun, you can imagine there will be a lot of drinking. Then of course there's a not-insignificant group of women who drink because the "excuse in a bottle," as Patrick puts it, gives them cover to act more

No one is drinking as much as you think they are.

uninhibitedly than they would if they were sober, especially when it comes to sex. We'll talk more about that soon, but it's an important factor to acknowledge when it comes to alcohol consumption in college.

A big part of the drinking-on-campus conversation that often gets overlooked is students who don't drink at all. Roughly a quarter of students on college campuses don't drink.[4] It's easy to imagine how alienated this group might feel, considering they, too, suffer from their peers' incorrectly estimating their numbers—college students guessed that only 5 percent of them never drink. If you truly believed you were in such a tiny minority, rather than a fairly sizable group, you might feel kind of down and out about your choices. But it doesn't have to be that way. Evelyn, nineteen, is a sophomore at a large university in the South who chooses not to drink. Aside from not being twenty-one yet, she has a lot of reasons for this choice—though to be clear, you don't need to rationalize choosing not to drink. For one, she's an engineering student, and as she puts it, "I like my brain a lot and I don't want to mess with it." This checks out, since early alcohol exposure in adolescents can negatively impact[5] learning and memory function in a developing brain. Second, both her parents struggled with alcoholism, and she doesn't want to see herself go down that path. Last, she tried it once or twice and just thinks it tastes gross, which is fair! A lot of alcohol tastes gross! Evelyn told me she doesn't experience a ton of one-on-one peer pressure to drink, but that the pressure comes more from society around her. It comes from the fact that there's a bar on her campus and that the weekend social scene at her school revolves around parties. Still, she doesn't let it stop her from participating. Evelyn told me she loves going to parties even though she's not drinking. All the things that everyone else is doing—dancing, flirting, talking—are still fun without a drink in her hand. Plus, she explains, she likes hanging out with drunk people to a point: They never look at her like she's nuts if she suggests going out for ice cream at 3 AM. When she's not being entertained by the antics of drunk friends, she fills her time with lots of activities, like a pole dancing aerobics class, which offers evening classes. Most important, she doesn't let being sober stop her from doing any of the things that are often associated with being drunk. Evelyn told me the story of the time she went to a Halloween party at a frat house. Halloween is widely considered to be one of the wilder party nights of the year, given the booze and skimpy costumes, but Evelyn had a goal. She just really wanted to make out with a stranger. A simple goal that might feel impossible without the "liquid courage" of a shot, but she sauntered up to a guy and did it nonetheless. She didn't need to be drunk to have fun and hook up, and neither do you.

PARTYING 201

Drink Smarter, Not Harder

Shocking as it is to hear, I, a semiprofessional adult, do think it's possible to mix booze, sex, and parties more or less safely. Why? Because it's happening all across the country at colleges every weekend. Yes, the risks are many and they are serious; no, you cannot control the actions of other people, but using responsible drinking strategies can greatly improve the quality of your experience and your overall safety. To learn how, I turned to Pritma "Mickey" Irizarry, director of the Health Promotion and Advocacy Center at American University in D.C.

There are a lot of choices you can make even before you start drinking that affect the type of night you'll have. The major outcome to avoid, Irizarry explains, is spiking your blood alcohol content (BAC) too quickly. Your BAC is a number that measures how much alcohol is in your bloodstream at a given time, and when that number rises quickly, you're more likely to experience negative side effects like throwing up or blacking out. To ensure that doesn't happen, start your night by eating a meal first. Another good backup strategy is to carry a substantial snack with you like a granola bar, in case your dinner wasn't quite enough. While Irizarry explains that food won't soak up the booze in your stomach and prevent you from getting drunk, it will slow down the rate that alcohol gets absorbed and potentially help you dodge some of those unpleasant outcomes. Also important to note when it comes to getting too messed up too fast? Mixing cannabis and alcohol can exacerbate the effects of both, potentially creating extra risk.

Another key component of what I like to think of as "defensive drinking" is being aware of how much alcohol you're consuming. This might seem like a, "well, duh," thing to say, but "one drink" is probably a lot less than you think it is. To test this theory, try and find a liquid measuring cup—like you'd use for cooking—and practice measuring standard drink sizes. Twelve ounces of beer might be easy to visualize because most of us are familiar with a standard soda can size, but if you measure out just 1.5 ounces (one standard drink in straight-shot form) or five ounces (one standard glass of wine), it's trickier to eyeball, and easier to overdo. Mixed drinks can get particularly risky. If you're pouring from a bottle rather than using a single shot glass to measure just 1.5 ounces, you can easily wind up with a cup that contains three or four drinks while thinking that this is your first drink of the night. Likewise, if you're filling a red Solo cup three quarters of the way with wine, it's more like two standard drinks.

Once you have a handle on what drink sizes actually look like, it's time to focus on how many of them you're having. The typical advice is to drink one standard drink an hour, two at most. And hey, if you're going to have that second drink, have a smaller serving of whatever it is and lower your risk of a BAC spike that way instead. Keeping a trained eye on how much you're drinking takes effort, and it might make you feel like a camp counselor, but you don't have to be conspicuous in order to take care of number one (that's you; you are always your first priority). If you've had your maximum amount of booze for the time being but don't want drunk partygoers obnoxiously asking you why you're not drinking, Irizarry suggests filling a cup with water or soda to get the bonus of extra hydration as well as something to do with your hands.

Here's what I do advocate when it comes to drinking games: cheating!

Now it's time to talk about two party staples that can derail your night from safe to scary: drinking games and shots. I will not look you in the eye and tell you never to partake in either! But it's not a secret that both activities lead to drinking a lot in a very short amount of time, which is a recipe for risk. So here's what I do advocate: cheating! If someone starts screaming, "Shots, shots, shots, shots, shots, shots, EVERYBODY!" and you've already had a drink or two in the last hour, you can still enjoy the party without pushing past your limits. Consider raising up your cup and taking a gulp of whatever is already in your hand to toast instead. Or, pour your shot yourself and just take a small splash instead of a full shot. Also: Beware double shot glasses! If the glassware at whatever party you wind up at looks taller or wider than a standard shot glass, don't fill it up all the way, because you might wind up drinking twice the amount you intended to.

When it comes to drinking games, especially games that require you to chug a drink, like Kings (my personal favorite back in the day, because

I loved the part where we all had to answer questions about which sex things each of us had done), just fake it. When someone pulled the card that signaled time for "waterfall," that is everybody chugging a drink in a circle until the first person stops, I would simply put my glass to my lips and pretend to be taking big, consecutive sips. In reality I was swallowing air. And if anyone ever calls you out for not following dumb, arbitrary game rules, I encourage you to borrow my line: "Oh, okay. Well, I can cheat, or I can chug this beer and throw up on your carpet. Which works better for you?"

Last up on your safe-drinking prep list is birth control. As the experts in this chapter have pointed out, a night of drinking can easily result in forgetting to take or use your birth control. If you're on birth control pills and you've realized that you keep forgetting it when you're partying on the weekends, consider moving the time of day you usually take it to dinner or even morning, so you'll be in a clear headspace when you do so. You've probably heard the tip to always carry condoms in your purse, which I fully endorse, but I like to go one step further. I'm willing to bet lots of you also keep condoms in a bedside table for easy access. If you're going out drinking and think there's even a tiny possibility that you might bring someone home, take a condom or two *out* of the drawer and put it on *top* of a night table or shelf before you leave. That way, when you come home, there will be a visual reminder to wrap it up, and you might be less likely to forget.

All told, knowing your limits boils down to a feeling more than a number, since different alcohols and amounts can affect people differently. If you're just starting to drink for the first time, try and do so in a small, controlled environment with people you trust. There's nothing wrong with a small dorm room gathering where you can really listen to your body without the risk of introducing strangers who might not have your best interests at heart.

BEYOND THE BASICS

When Your Drinking Becomes an Excuse

It's been well documented by writers and researchers alike that some young women report feeling like they need alcohol in order to be sexually intimate with a partner, especially a new one. My conversations with current college students did little to buck the trend, and I saw two groups emerge: those who drank because sex itself felt uncomfortable or awkward without booze, and those who drank because they were self-conscious about their bodies and what their partners would think of them. It goes without saying there was certainly some overlap between these groups. Women: Our anxieties contain multitudes!

Lisa, who goes to school in North Carolina, estimates that about 70 percent of her hookups are preceded by alcohol. "It takes away the pressure to be good enough," she says. When I press her to explain what the pressure was, she lists several dynamics booze made her forget about: how her hair looked, how her body looked, if her performance was good enough. She acknowledges that heavy drinking at parties led to some behaviors she didn't like, such as guys grabbing her inappropriately, feigning that they just needed to scoot her aside to pass by. Still, she insists, drinking makes you happy, which was a benefit that could lead to, or at least help, hookups in her mind.

Which takes us back to alcohol expectancy theory. If you believe booze paves the way for a hookup, it may start occurring that way, but that doesn't mean it's actually the alcohol that's doing the work. In fact, I'd argue alcohol can actually make sex markedly worse. You've heard the term "whiskey dick," when being drunk can make it hard to maintain an erection, but my experts also pointed out that alcohol can make it more challenging for women to climax, as well. Not to mention, being drunk can mess with your ability to communicate, which can also make it more challenging to have fulfilling sex. Therein lies the problem with getting too drunk and getting consent. The initial conversation of "Do I want to be sexually intimate with this person?" might be easy, but consent is a moving needle that needs to be constantly reassessed as sex is happening, and alcohol can make picking up on body language or expressing your feelings impossibly hard. I wish I had a handy tip for this one, but I don't. You can make lists in your phone of all the people at any given party you'd like to sleep with when you arrive, so that later, when you're a bit more drunk, you already have an innate sense of who you wanted to go home with—and who didn't make the pre-approved list. You can tell your friends that you're not looking to hook up tonight at all. But once you're home with a partner, those same issues will arise. The best way to keep a clear head is to always aim to be in the tipsy-drunk headspace, rather than drunk-drunk.

Leah, who just graduated from a large university in Pennsylvania, has a problem that's not at all uncommon: Although she's been sexually active since she was in high school, she tells me she's never had a sober sexual experience. Leah explains that due in part to a sexual assault in her teen years and conflict in her parents' marriage, she has an extremely difficult time trusting partners, which she connects with her drinking habits. Leah wouldn't be considered an alcoholic by any measure, but she relies on drinking until she feels a buzz to stem her anxieties surrounding sex. Her fears are all too relatable: She worries about what her body looks like, if she's making funny faces, what her partner thinks about her vagina, and so on. She understands it's an unhealthy crutch, she knows the booze impedes her ability to orgasm, and she knows her fears aren't based in truth (to date, no one has left her bed due to funny sex face!), but she cannot fathom sex without alcohol. When I asked her to picture sober sex and what that might be like for her, I can practically hear her recoiling, as she let out a string of "No, no, no, no!"

"I couldn't even imagine it," she tells me. She wants to believe that with the right partner who could accept her anxieties, she'd be able to have substance-free intimacy, but she hasn't reached that point yet, even with partners she's been seeing on and off for months. And although a shot or two gives Leah the ability to let her guard down enough to participate in sex, she recognizes it comes with its own drawbacks as well, like agreeing to certain things in bed or partners she wouldn't have sober. She has a hard time saying no, she tells me. Leah's raw honesty is at once refreshing and a little heartbreaking. Refreshing, because she shares with pride that she's actively working on her underlying issues with a therapist, which is a crucial step to take if you discover you've become reliant on any substance. But heartbreaking because I relate to her deeply. I went through a phase in college where I had sex with just about everyone who showed interest in me because I was addicted to the high of being wanted. When your self-esteem is low and you're not feeling pride or approval from other areas of your life, the feeling of someone desiring you is a hard habit to kick.

But if you're willing to do the hard work, ideally with a trained professional, you can. Dr. Rachel Needle, a licensed psychologist and sex therapist whom I spoke with, echoes the familiar theme that many of us are raised with a lack of education that breeds general misunderstanding when it comes to sex. But beyond that, becoming booze-reliant for sex could mean that you're acting in a way that's fundamentally misaligned with your sexual values.

Your sexual values, Dr. Needle explained to me, are your core set of beliefs about sex. And even though "value" sounds like an inherently positive thing, it's possible to hold lots of unhealthy sexual values. For example, if you were raised to believe that anyone who has sex before marriage is an awful person, it's not surprising that you might turn to alcohol or drugs beforehand to help you dissociate that behavior from the rigid, punishing idea that what you're doing is fundamentally wrong.

If you want to dive deeper, Needle suggests interrogating your own set of sexual values. Try opening up a journal and splitting a page into two columns. On one side, list as many things you believe about sex as you can. Such as, "I believe both partners should be responsible for contraception," or "You shouldn't have sex until the third hookup," or "Reverse cowgirl is an overrated position." For each belief, ask yourself: Is this something I believe or is this something someone told me? When did I first learn this? Is this based on my own experience or someone else's? Do I still believe this is true, or have I changed my mind? Record your corresponding analysis for each point in the second column. You might be surprised to find that something you took for granted when you were younger doesn't feel right to you anymore as a young adult.

Ultimately, by deconstructing the tapestry of facts and opinions that make up your values, you may be able to rewrite them into a set of conduct that feels authentic to you, and that you don't have to hide from with booze. Another method to delve deeper into your inhibitions, Needle explains, is practicing mindfulness. If the stress of your body and your performance overwhelms you to the point of needing to dampen and hide from those feelings with alcohol, try some mindfulness exercises. Many free or cheap meditation apps can walk you through it. Practicing being fully in the moment for things that are entirely unrelated to sex (think: When you're eating, be aware of how each bite of food feels and tastes in your mouth, stop to feel the sensation of chewing, and fully focus your mind on that one task at hand) can help you be more present when the time comes to get it on. Give yourself permission to feel all the feelings associated with a certain act, let the bad ones like guilt or embarrassment roll off after you acknowledge them, and concentrate on the things that are happening in the moment that make you feel good. After a while, the things that initially worried you might start to weigh a little less heavily on your mind.

⚠️ **Don't ignore the voices in your head that tell you *I need this drink* before sex. If it happens more often than not, and you truly can't enjoy intimacy when you're sober, it's time to reach out for some help.**

ℓℓℓℓ

Today, when my social life revolves less around bars and more around a glass of red wine with a late-night deadline, or taking advantage of an open bar at my friends' weddings, I've realized I drink a lot less than I did when I was twenty-two. It doesn't mean I don't still have one too many martinis and wake up with an olive brine–induced headache, or take a shot and make the craziest dancing faces to ever wind up in a wedding album, but the difference is that I feel like I'm fun to be around whether I'm drinking or not. And that translates to sex, too. Do I occasionally reach for a weed gummy if I'm having a stressful day and need to leave my racing thoughts behind? You bet—it's legal in my home state of California and it helps me feel more aware of myself during sex. But with time, trial and error, and rehashing mistakes, I've found a balance between being buzzed and just being me.

4.

Taking Your Time

I Promise, You're Not the Only One Not Having Sex

I was eating lunch in my high school cafeteria when I first discovered that someone I actually knew had had sex. We were sophomores, and none of us had "done it" yet, so my friends and I sat, rapt, as this girl we knew nonchalantly divulged that she and her older boyfriend had recently gotten busy. We threw around dated (and in retrospect, harmful) euphemisms like "punching your v-card" and "giving it up" as we begged for details. Nowadays, I don't even like to use the phrase "losing your virginity," but we'll get into that a bit later. I was struck by how mature and confident this girl now seemed, our tour guide returning from the vast horny unknown, charting points of interest on the map of our uncertainty. I couldn't shake how childish I felt around her all of a sudden. No one else I knew was sexually active, besides the odd hand job here and there, but even so, I had a powerful feeling that there was some VIP sex club I didn't have access to. For a young person to feel immature, left out, delayed, or like a"prude" is a dangerous combination that can blind you to reality and make you feel like time is ticking on your sexual debut, when that couldn't be further from the truth.

It's a fact that can't be proven until you actually experience it, but having sex for the first doesn't fundamentally alter you in any way. You will be no different. Your hair won't be shinier, your skin won't be clearer, you won't be more mature. The only thing you'll know that you didn't before is what someone's mouth and/or genitals feel like in/on your mouth/genitals. That's it! It's practically worthy of a novelty mug that reads "I had sex, and all I got was this tiny bit of trivia." This isn't to say it can't be exciting, meaningful, loving, passionate, hot, and scary all at once, but if you're turning to sex and thinking it's going to transform you and your relationship in a massive way, it likely won't. After I had intercourse for the first time, an overall neutral-to-positive experience, I was shocked at the nothingness of it all. This doesn't mean I didn't like it or that my partner wasn't kind and responsive, but it felt so anticlimactic as it was occurring that I vividly recall thinking as I lay prone on a bunk bed in Seattle, "Wait, is this it?" And this is why I don't like the term "losing your virginity." As crucial as it is to realize you don't necessarily gain anything from a first-time experience, it's doubly so to remember that you *lose* absolutely nothing once you become

> **You are still you, no matter what you do when you're naked.**

sexually active. No magical piece of you drifts away, you don't get a punch on a card that gets you closer to a free sandwich. You are still just the same—and that's a wonderful thing. Even the term *virgin*, trying to delineate some tangible difference between those who have sex and those who don't, becomes meaningless when you affirm to yourself that you are still you, no matter what you do when you're naked.

But I didn't have to tackle these feelings when I was in college, a time when, statistically, the older you get, the more likely[1] you are to be sexually active. So I talked to young women and experts alike about how to tamp down the ticking of that imaginary clock, whether you're consciously choosing not to have sex or it just hasn't happened yet.

WE'RE ALL HAVING LESS SEX THAN YOU THINK

While there are lots of contributing factors, experts agree: We're having less sex than in decades past. Whereas 51 percent of sexually active people were having sex once or more a week in 1996, now we're clocking in at 39 percent.[2] And there are more young adults than ever who report never having had sex.[3] Sure, these facts alone might sound concerning to some: What if we go into a birthrate decline so sharp that the population whittles away to nothing? Does this mean we're all perpetually miserable and starved for intimacy? There's more going on than meets the eye, and more than a smidgeon of hope. Debby Herbenick, PhD, a professor at Indiana University's School of Public Health, has been one of the researchers pointing out the potential good in this decline. For one, she told me, nowadays there's less alcohol use than in decades past, so it could be that there's less drunken sex occurring, which, if you were paying attention to the last chapter, you know isn't the worst thing to cut down on. She adds, anecdotally, that more and more of her students have shared that they just want to wait until the conditions are right for the type of sex *they* want to have, rather than going with the flow of hookup culture and getting naked with someone just because they're hot and at the same party. I'll note that there's absolutely nothing wrong with doing that if you *want* to, but being able to separate what you *want* to be doing from what you think you *should* be doing is a skill worth celebrating. Another possible factor behind the sex slowdown? After the Obama administration's focus on campus sexual assault (not to mention the reckoning of the #MeToo movement), people are being more thoughtful about how they approach sex and consent to avoid harming themselves or their partners.

While this sex recession sometimes gets blamed on smartphones (and sure, social media use has been known to increase anxiety, which is on the rise, and anxiety doesn't help our sex drives[4]) by now it's clear that's too simplistic of a scapegoat. Your phone isn't single-handedly going to lower the American birth rate and cause the downfall of society all on its own. But just because we can debunk one myth, that doesn't mean all the sex trends researchers are looking at paint a rosy picture, either. Herbenick's research has also noted an increase in rough sex behaviors like choking without prior discussion. While this hunch hasn't yet been studied, Herbenick suggests there could be a correlation there. "I do have to wonder," she muses, "if that's been your experience, how likely are you to want to hook up with somebody again if the last time you did, somebody squeezed your neck?"

Ultimately, Herbenick also advises looking back in time to when we *were* having more sex. The statistics that some researchers are holding up are from a time when marital rape was legal and drunk driving (and therefore more drunk and potentially coercive sex) was the norm. By comparison, this sex slowdown could, in fact, be a very good thing. And finally, when all else fails, stop comparing altogether. Herbenick offers a much more helpful rubric. "Ask yourself, 'Am I happy with the sex life that I have? What do I want to change to feel better about it?'" she explains. "Those are much more important questions than 'Have I had sex yet or not?'"

SEX FOMO 101

What We Mean When We Say "Sex"

If you're concerned that you're not having sex, part of that anxiety could be, in part, because of how we're defining it. Well-regarded sex educator Al Vernacchio explained to me that if we could look at sex through the lens of a whole set of behaviors and actions, rather than a boiled-down version of "part A goes into part B," we'd have a much healthier mindset. For example, if you say sex has to be intimate, consensual, pleasurable, and enthusiastic for it to really be sex, we wouldn't all be so focused on vaginal intercourse as the be-all and end-all. Having anal sex or oral sex isn't any lower down on the sex totem pole: All of these activities, and others I haven't even thought of, "count" just as much. You may be sexually active and already participating in the erotic buffet of life without even realizing it (and without enjoying it to the fullest!) if you consider yourself a "virgin" just because you haven't had a penetrative experience. You don't need to put that stress on yourself when there are so many ways to be sexual with a partner. Think: masturbating near each other, stimulating each other manually, deep kissing, full-naked body contact *while* you kiss deeply, using vibrators, etc. Not to mention, a view of "sex = intercourse" largely erases the experience of queer people, who may choose penetrative activities involving a toy, a hand, or even none at all! Sex is valid without a penis, thank you very much. And finally, on a bittersweet note, Vernacchio says he often gets asked by young women, "Am I still a virgin if I've been sexually assaulted?" While there's little one can say or do to erase that kind of trauma, a more inclusive view of sex can render that question unnecessary and ease the burden just a little. Rape isn't consensual, and therefore rape isn't sex.

Opening up our definitions and understanding can have a whole world of unexpected benefits.

The Waiting Game

Expanding your personal definition of what sex means is a lot easier said than done, I get it. You can't just snap your fingers and wish your anxieties away—if you could, my therapist would be out of a job. No one understands that better than Priya, a senior at a large university in the Northeast. Although she's had oral sex, Priya is apprehensive about never having had intercourse. She grew up being able to talk about sex freely and her friends at college maintain what feels like almost comical sex positivity, and I mean that in the kindest of ways. "We'll text each other and be like, 'Don't come to my room, I'm masturbating now!,'" she tells me. In this way, Priya is the perfect example of what it means to understand something intellectually, but not always be able to carry it out in practice. "I think because it feels [like everyone's having sex], it's harder for me to do it now. Because the older I get, it feels like there's more of a gap," she explains. And she's nervous for people to know. As a result, when social conversations turn to sex, she plays up the experience she *has* had, to try and conceal her insecurity. Priya has done a remarkable amount of introspection to try and unpack her complicated feelings. For one, she knows that she's extremely self-conscious about her body, which makes it hard for her to get intimate with people. Priya, a woman of color, went to a mostly white high school, where people made offhand, derogatory comments about her skin. On top of that, her parents put a lot of pressure on her to lose weight when she was young. Understandably, if you've been made to feel bad about your body, showing it to people can feel shameful, if not impossible. When she tries to date, she often encounters other roadblocks: for one, racial fetishizers. She vividly recalls briefly seeing a guy, who, after it didn't work out between the two of them, paraded across campus with a stream of other women who looked exactly like her. And for another, virgin fetishizers. On the rare occasion she does tell people she's never had intercourse, she'll sometimes get the reaction "Oh, that's hot."

⚠ In case it's not apparent why that's a red flag, anyone who is actively turned on by virginity, by the prospect of being the "first" to "take" something from you, who believes someone who's never had sex is more valuable or attractive than those who have, is probably not a super great person!

Priya often struggles with a particular question, one that she assumes others must wonder about her, which is "Why, in your early twenties, haven't you done this yet?" The irrational part of her assumes it must be because she, or anyone in her position, is undesirable or socially awkward. So I asked her to answer that question for herself. Why haven't you? For Priya, it boils down to fear and insecurity, two totally normal emotions that have nothing to do with her inherent value as a person. So, if that's a question you're worried about, genuinely answer it for yourself. The answer probably isn't as scary as you think. It can be anything, including fear, just not wanting to, not having had the right opportunity, concerns about pregnancy, or any number of mind-numbingly average, completely relatable reasons. None of which signal that there's anything wrong with you. Another piece of advice Priya gave herself is to actively work on her own insecurity; she and her friends made a pact for her to go on a couple of Tinder or Bumble dates a week, even just to talk to people, to slowly up her comfort level for eventual intimate exchanges.

Ultimately, those who aren't having sex, especially those who are not actively choosing not to, might find comfort in data.[5] If you're of the mindset that literally everyone is having sex except you, you might be surprised to know that 36.5 percent of college students have never had vaginal intercourse. Roughly 35 percent haven't had any sexual partners in the last twelve months, and 40.2 percent have had just one partner in the past twelve months. That is far from the all-weekend fuck-fest many of us consider college to be. Carolyn, a freshman at a medium-sized university in Texas, is someone who, beyond the data, takes comfort in knowing she's not alone in her choice not to have sex. In fact, she's part of a religious-based sorority, and having the support of her sisters makes her feel even more secure in her beliefs. Carolyn isn't of the mindset that having sex before marriage is some kind of sin that damns you to hell; she just wants to be in a long-term relationship that she sees a future in, where she feels support without any pressure to move faster than she wants to. She doesn't feel left out of the party scene at her school at all either, because she's met some interesting people that way—just no love connections yet. After all, not having sex doesn't mean not dating. Carolyn uses dating apps, too, with mixed results. While most people are respectful when she tells them she's not in this for sex, she has matched with a handful of guys who've gotten angry. She's sometimes met with comments like, "You're missing out!" or "Why do you have to be like that?" or, my personal favorite, "I can show you all this fun stuff." This is just one woman's opinion here, but when a guy starts trying to coax you on a magic carpet ride, you almost certainly don't need what he's selling. Carolyn's main piece of advice for others is just to be calm but direct with people about where you're at. She says things like, "I'm not about that," or "That's not what I'm looking for," and keeps the conversation light. The experts I spoke to agree it's good to let people know these kinds of things up-front, because we all deserve to find what we're looking for in a partnership, and no one wants to be surprised with a potential deal breaker late in the game. Most important, she understands there's no one-size-fits-all advice when it comes to sex and doesn't judge what anyone else decides to do. "I'm not trying to shame anyone for doing that, it's just something that I chose not to do," Carolyn explains. "If you, partake, you partake!" she added with a giggle.

When I was in college, I never stopped to consider how varied the factors are behind young adults' not having sex. For example, Amy, a junior at a university in St. Louis, Missouri, identifies as asexual. If that term is new to you, Amy explains that it basically means she doesn't experience sexual attraction. She just never saw the appeal of hooking up. Amy was in high school when she first realized people were pairing off and couldn't understand what the big deal was. Her understanding of her identity grew from there, and in college, it presented challenges to building relationships of all sorts. She's had friends blow off plans with her to go hook up with guys, which is a complicated betrayal for Amy. "I was kind of getting kicked to the curb for something, and I didn't even understand why [my friend] wanted it," she says. She does want a relationship, and she knows if she made a Tinder and put "ace" (shorthand for asexual) in her bio, she might have a better chance of finding one. But she's resistant to the idea, and it's hard for her to pinpoint why. Just because certain technology exists doesn't mean everyone is comfortable using it, which is especially difficult for marginalized communities that tend to thrive within online communities. Even though Amy hasn't found the type of platonic boyfriend she'd like to have, she's developed an incredible group of peers who she "stays up watching movies until 4 AM with." She doesn't feel like she's missing out at all and has some useful advice for anyone in her shoes looking to build a community that doesn't revolve around who you're going home with that night: "Be yourself in a public setting or open setting," Amy says. After all, she grew her current gang of friends by reading or watching TV in common rooms, which attracted like-minded people to her. If you broadcast who you are and what you want, you give others a chance to find you.

There could be groups of people, too, who are less likely to join in the hookup scene, and privilege plays a role. Shemeka Thorpe, PhD, a sexuality researcher and cofounder of The Minority Sex Report, whose work focuses on Black and Native American women, points out that first-generation college students may have fewer partners on campus, too. She explains that from her personal experience and research, first-generation college students may be more likely to be sexually active with someone they know from back home or they're in a long-term relationship with, than they are to be engaged in casual sex. There are a bunch of reasons, she's learned, that "for first-generation students, college itself can sometimes be intimidating. You're trying to navi-

Just because you've *been* sexually active, it doesn't mean you need to *keep* being sexually active if it's not working for you.

gate a space where your family or maybe even your friends have never navigated, so you're focused on that academically. There's sometimes a fear that you can't mess up or get distracted because you're the only person in your family to go." And so, the privilege of hooking up freely isn't something they necessarily get, and they may be more comfortable going back to a familiar partner who they've known longer. Thorpe adds that some of these students may be from lower-income families and working jobs as well, and they may not have the time to go out and engage in the kind of activities that lead to casual sex.

Then there's Erika, a junior at UCLA, who was dating someone from high school but broke up with him her sophomore year of college. She hasn't had sex in about a year, and has no plans to start up again anytime soon. As a newly single person, Erika says she felt some pressure from her friends to "get back out there" and to get over her ex by getting under someone else. A part of her agreed, but ultimately, she just didn't want to. Erika had spent a lot of time teaching her ex about what she liked, and she'd heard lots of stories from her friends of painfully awkward and unfulfilling hookups. As a result, she wasn't eager to go from the comfort of someone who knew her body well to hookups that largely leave women much less satisfied than men. Data suggests that in a first-time casual hookup, men will orgasm 31 percent of the time, while women do just 11 percent of the time.[6] While an orgasm isn't the only metric for satisfaction, it's certainly a part of it. "I just don't want to deal with shitty sex," she tells me. Eventually, she figured out she doesn't have to. Just because you've *been* sexually active, it doesn't mean you need to *keep* being sexually active if it's not working for you. "Once that switch of starting to have sex is flipped on, there's this idea that it needs to keep going. I think that's a pressure I didn't realize I was feeling. It's almost like once you discover the magic of sex and how great it can be that you need to keep experiencing it and liberate yourself. But I'm liberating myself by choosing not to as well." So when her body is telling her to go out and run toward the first available penis she can find, but her brain doesn't want to, Erika masturbates instead. (Hey, it's good advice in just about any situation). Erika learned that a sex hiatus is just fine with her for the time being, and slowly but surely, her friends got it, too.

SEX FOR NEWBIES 201

Getting Ready

Even though this is a chapter about *not* having sex, some of you may decide to start at some point in college. And even when your body and brain slowly start aligning to send you the "ALL SYSTEMS GO (DOWN)!" signal, you may still be wondering if you're actually ready. To help clear up some lingering doubts, Al Vernacchio, Shemeka Thorpe, and I chipped in some of our favorite considerations for you to ponder beforehand.

The Am I Ready For This? Checklist

DO I TRUST THIS PARTNER?

You hear a lot about love being the major prerequisite for sex, but trust—the ability to believe a partner when they share their STI status, to put faith in their capacity to care for you and treat you with empathy—might matter even more.

COULD I HAVE SEX SOBER AND WITH THE LIGHTS ON?

Being nervous or insecure is completely normal, especially for a first time with a new partner. But if you're relying on crutches to hide from facing that discomfort, you might not be quite ready.

DO I KNOW WHAT I LIKE, AND COULD I EXPLAIN THAT TO A PARTNER?

In order to be able to have sex, any kind of sex, you need to be able to talk about it. Otherwise, you risk being in a situation where you're handing over all your power and control because you're too nervous to speak up. While absolutely no one expects you to be able to describe your ideal intimate experience like you're reading it from a car owner's manual, you should have explored and experimented enough on your own that you can give a little guidance.

DO I HAVE A GAME PLAN FOR MY MEDICAL CARE?

Just like you need to be able to communicate with a partner, you should also be comfortable talking about sex with your doctor. Once you become sexually active, you'll need to know where to go to get testing, birth control, routine exams, and more. Do a little research about the closest clinics beforehand so that you're not scrambling to figure it all out after.

This is a nonexhaustive list, but being honest with yourself about some of the most important pre-sex questions can make listening to your gut a little easier.

Let's Talk About (Talking About) First-Time Sex, Baby

Once you think you might be ready, or even if you're still figuring it out, keeping an open line of communication with that potential first partner is important. But, if you've never done something before, talking about it may not come naturally. Just as with every sex conundrum you're likely to face, we've got a plan for that!

While you may be picturing this as one big sex talk, Thorpe recommends breaking it down into a few conversations. The first time you bring it up, try simply sharing that you've never done XYZ activity before. Maybe with the second conversation, you can talk about what kind of birth control you might be using, or STI statuses, then perhaps share something you like in bed, and so on. The idea here is simple but effective: You don't need to hype yourself up for one big "I'm ready!!!!!" disclosure. These types of bite-size information can be shared in small talk. In a perfect world, we'd have all these conversations with our clothes still on, when sex is a hypothetical and not an inevitability. But Thorpe understands that the world isn't perfect, so if you've had some of these Hansel and Gretel breadcrumb–type conversations, you've laid some healthy groundwork already, just in case you do get caught up in a sexy, spontaneous moment.

Vernacchio suggests that no matter how you decide to talk about it, make verbal choices that add to your feeling of empowerment. Let a potential partner know this is new to you, but that you feel comfortable with them and you've made the choice to experience it with them. As Vernacchio puts it, "Rather than 'I'm gonna let you do this to me,' it's 'I'm choosing you as my partner in this moment.'" That's part of the reason it's so important to understand your own body, too. Some people may assume a person who hasn't been sexually active has no idea what to do and therefore they should just take the lead instead. You can disabuse someone of that notion by walking in armed with knowledge and declare, "Hey, I haven't done this particular thing before, but I really love kisses on my neck and quick taps on my clit." You are the expert on you, always.

Finally, it may surprise you to hear this, but there is absolutely no moral imperative to share that it's your first time. But! This free pass comes with a caveat: Just because you don't necessarily have to disclose that fact doesn't mean there aren't potential benefits to doing so. For one, it could take some pressure off you to perform "perfectly" your first time. For another, most decent humans would want to take things even more slowly and deliberately, knowing it was their partner's first time. But, as my sources have explained, if the stress of sharing that particular fact adds so much anxiety that it begins to detract from the overall positivity of the experience, no one is twisting your arm here. Provided you feel confident in understanding and communicating about your body, you should make the choices that render you the most in control and relaxed you can possibly be.

ℓℓℓℓ

Having sex doesn't give you magic powers or make you cooler than your friends, but it can leave you feeling disappointed if you're buying into outdated myths. I wish I'd known just how many people my age *weren't* having sex at school. I wish I'd known that I could simply stop seeking out new partners once I started and it didn't mean I was in a "dry spell." But mostly, I wish I had more nonjudgmental people to talk to about all the weird feelings that my first time evoked. I think back to that bunk bed in Seattle, barely even understanding how intercourse was supposed to work. I dabbed myself with toilet paper in the bathroom afterward, and even cried for a minute when I saw a few faint drops of blood. Still, I don't regret it. I don't regret it because I made the choice to do it with someone I trusted, no one pressured me into it, and I dictated the terms myself. Even if your first time "story" is incredibly unromantic; even if your primary motivation is just curiosity, if you have the right foundation and faith in your choices, you're setting yourself up for a lifetime of sexual experiences that, cumulatively, will teach you so much more about yourself than one "first" ever could.

5.

I've Got a Vibrator and I'm Not Afraid to Use It

Learning and Asking for What You Really Want in Bed

My very first vibrator was a birthday gift from my ninth-grade boyfriend. Yes, I know: This is not the typical sex-toy origin story, but stick with me. I had recently started running, and after sharing with him that my legs were feeling sore as a result, he purchased what he believed to be a muscle massager. While he had no idea the small, oblong device was likely intended for stimulating more than just muscles, he presented it to me with pride. In all fairness, I had no idea what it was either, but it certainly helped with my aching quads. And then I decided I was over running, and it sat in my bedside table drawer for a year. I can't remember when, why, or how it dawned on me to revisit it one afternoon, but that day I learned something I'd spend the next ten years ignoring: I can, with few exceptions, only orgasm if I'm using a vibrator. Even typing that sentence, as a woman in my thirties, brings a flush of embarrassment. Every single

> **When it comes to what you like, there is no normal. There is only "what works for me."**

gle insecure, paranoid thought I used to worry my past partners might think about me, I've now begun to worry that you, reading this, might think too: *What if they think I'm weird? What if they think I'm broken? Am I broken? Does it mean I'm bad at masturbating? Does it mean I'm bad at sex?*

For those reasons and so many more, I rarely shared the one, tiny, buzzy addition that could have made dozens of sexual encounters way better for me. I prioritized having sex; I didn't prioritize having good-for-me sex. I wanted to feel attractive above all else, and I didn't place a premium on feeling heard or having my needs met. When you think about sex as it is portrayed in movies, TV, and even porn, you rarely see someone grabbing for a condom or talking about testing, let alone reaching into their drawer to get their vibrator. So I hardly ever brought it up, because I didn't want to ruin the fantasy my partners might have had. I didn't want to do anything during sex that I didn't see as normal. What I didn't realize then is that when it comes to what you like, there is no normal. There is only "what works for me," and by being too scared to share some harmless facts about how my body works, I was hiding from myself and denying my partners the chance to genuinely make me feel the best I possibly could. And guess what? Of the handful of boyfriends or hookups I *did* tell, not one guy made me feel any of those scary feelings I worried about. To my knowledge, there were no rumors floating around the campus center about the sex freak who can't come without a battery. No guys ever ran screaming from my dorm.

It's honestly a little depressing to think about all the orgasms I've lost out on over the years, yet it underscores just how difficult it is to communicate about pleasure. But it doesn't have to be.

THAT'S WHAT I WANT 101

Why It Feels So Hard to Communicate about Sex

I don't blame myself for not speaking up with each and every partner I've had. To do so would be to ignore the ways the deck has been stacked against people socialized as women. Dr. Sandra Byers, a professor of psychology at the University of New Brunswick and a licensed clinical psychologist who I spoke to, explains that there are several harmful myths that affect the ways we talk, or don't talk, about our own pleasure. For one, there's the sexist notion that women mainly pursue sex for the relationship that may result from it, whereas men are just in it for the sex. While this totally erases the multitudes of women who enjoy casual sex, it also reinforces the idea that if you're a woman and you want to keep this hypothetical guy around, you shouldn't rock the boat by suggesting you might want things your partner isn't delivering, otherwise he won't ever be your boyfriend. This, obviously, is bullshit. If you grew up hearing this myth and therefore assumed that sex was the best way to get a potential boyfriend to commit, you'd probably be a lot less likely to advocate for yourself.

Then there's the myth of the mind reader. Byers explains that all too often, we expect our partners to know exactly what we want in bed, and if they do not, it's somehow a judgment on us and the relationship. We falsely assume we're less in tune with each other if we can't magically produce orgasms on demand without any guidance. But talking about what you want and need beforehand doesn't make the resulting sex any less valid. Buying into this myth has created a false image of what it means to be "good in bed": someone who can play your body like a violin while you just lie back, appreciating it in silent reverie. And like . . . sure. That would be great. But it's unrealistic and puts an incredible amount of pressure on your partner. Too often, men are also negatively impacted by the notion that they're supposed to be sex gurus who know everything there is to know about vaginas. The reality is, a good lover isn't a sex psychic. A good lover is a good teacher and a good listener.

Last, this kind of communication doesn't get modeled for young adults nearly enough. Not only have I never seen a realistic portrayal of someone bringing their vibrator into bed with a partner, but similarly, depictions of someone verbally guiding their partner with precise and positive reinforcement are also rare. Mainstream images of sex are typically split into awkward fumbling for comedic effect, or the dramatic, seamless merging of bodies without a word between them, save a breathy moan of pleasure. Neither does much to help mirror the ways we can explain our preferences to our partners. Byers adds that parents don't always model communication well either. It's easy to talk to your kid about the difference between good touches and bad touches, or instill that yes means yes and no means no, but oftentimes parents are wholly out of their league when it comes to helping their daughter explain how she likes her clitoris touched. For the record, I absolutely would not have responded well to any such conversation, had my parents tried to broach the topic. But it just goes to further underscore how woefully short of positive modeling we are when it comes to pleasure.

The Inequity of Pleasure

We're all pretty bad at communicating about sex. One study of couples showed that on average, even after dating for fourteen years, partners still hadn't told each other everything about their sexual desires.[1] Can you imagine being with one person for more than a decade but still not sharing all the things you want in bed? I can, because lots of women, even today, are socialized to be people pleasers, and that can prevent honest communication when it comes to sex. Still, it's important to acknowledge and understand that, yes, women might have a tougher time than men expressing their needs as a group, and for queer women and women of color, this might present even more of a challenge. Gaining perspective on how our intersecting identities and specific upbringings compound difficulties surrounding sex is critical to understanding where we go from here.

Across the board, women of color and queer women are more at risk for domestic violence. Understandably, people experiencing abuse can feel silenced by that trauma both now and in the future. But it goes further than that: Women who don't fit conventional standards of beauty, be it body shape or disability, might also share that sense of being silenced. When you're given the message over and over again that you're not good enough, that you don't measure up, it makes it harder to believe in your inherent worth. This narrative pushes women to settle for whatever they can get, which can translate to not advocating for yourself both in bed and in the relationship itself, a dangerous path to go down.

Then, consider those who experience sexual pain. While there is a range of causes for painful sex, like vaginismus, vulvodynia, or pelvic floor dysfunction, there's a common thread: Sexual pain often takes several years to diagnose. Too often women with these conditions are dismissed and told they're just nervous, or that sex is supposed to hurt. If you've been conditioned to think sex ought to be painful, you're less likely to seek care or speak up.

Add to that people who may not have grown up with any sex ed, especially those in rural communities without the same access to resources like free clinics that those in more urban areas may have. Or queer people who got sex ed that didn't address their ways of intimacy at all. The sum of this disheartening calculus gives us tons of people who don't even have the language to discuss sex beyond the basics of intercourse. All of this matters, because without detangling the ways in which women, and certain communities within that group, have been screwed over into silence, we can't hope to break the pattern.

STUDYING YOUR BODY 201
Break Out the Basics

If you are going to smash the cycle that all too often leaves women suffering through bad sex, you have to start with figuring out what you like yourself. This is crucial. If you can't figure out what gives you pleasure on your own, how can you explain it to someone else? Justine Ang Fonte, MEd, MPH, a New York City sex educator who works with K–12 schools across the United States, advises starting with a bit of advice you've probably heard before: Get a mirror, and examine your vagina. Cliché, right? Maybe, but have you ever thought about why we're told to do this? It's not because it's some Judy Blume–esque rite of passage, or because the beauty of our own genitalia is so arresting it moves us to tears (although if the latter is the case for you, all the more power to you!). It comes from the simple sentiment that knowledge is power. By now you've probably heard that the clitoris, the small nub where the labia meet, is the pleasure center for most women, and likely your best bet for an orgasm. But, as Fonte explains, "If you didn't even know that you had a clitoris, you'd probably never use it. If you learned that there *is* a clitoris and what it does, you need to know where it is so that you can activate it." You cannot give yourself pleasure without understanding the parts of your body and what they do. You can't easily explain how someone else can give you pleasure if you don't know how to name those parts. Suddenly, what seems like a cliché, a bit of advice whispered between women before they flee into bathrooms with makeup compact mirrors, becomes the immutable foundation of pleasure.

What is really at stake when we don't know ourselves intimately? We lower the bar for what we accept, sometimes to dangerous ends. Katie, a junior at a university in the South, started using Tinder and dating when she was twenty. Her first sexual encounter, she explains, wasn't a positive one. While she had experimented a bit with masturbating, she felt completely in the dark when she found herself in her date's bedroom one night. "I really didn't know what I enjoyed until I started being sexually active," she tells me. And while it's true that partners can introduce us to a lot of new things that feel good, we can't rely on them to do everything for us. Katie's first partner didn't care very much about how she felt, and she had a hard time calling him out on it. "I never communicated with him because I didn't know what I was doing. So I just let him take the reins," she says. She was afraid to tell him that it was her first time. Once they started having sex that night, he warned her to be quiet so others in the house wouldn't hear them. Then, hardly a moment later, he grabbed a pillow from the other side of the bed and

Start with figuring out what you like.

put it on her face to muffle any sounds. Not knowing what to do, Katie held it there until he had orgasmed and the sex stopped. Looking back on it now, she felt objectified, and from the tone of her voice, I'd guess still pretty hurt, too. But she didn't speak up in the moment. "I think there was a lot of pressure," Katie explains. "I guess I didn't want to ruin the moment for him. And in my head I'm thinking, 'This guy likes me.' I just didn't want to ruin anything and I don't know why, because there was nothing to ruin." These experiences can be formative in such a damaging way. Imagine thinking this is normal behavior from a partner: You might go on allowing this for the rest of your life. Thankfully, Katie took this experience and demanded more from the next person she dated. She told him right off the bat that she didn't have a lot of experience, she wanted to go slow, and he easily accepted that information. Now, instead of being too scared to share what's going on, they can talk openly and honestly about what they like and don't like in bed.

Once you have a sense of your body (hint: You can accurately locate your labia, vulva, clitoris, and feel the entrance to your vaginal canal, to start), it's time to start figuring out what you like. Fonte explains it's important to think about how your body receives sensation, even if it's not in a sexual context. Really start paying attention to how it feels when you insert a tampon, for example. Is it different, better, or worse if you use a menstrual cup, for example? How does it feel when you have pubic hair, versus if you remove it? All these exercises help you get comfortable with identifying pleasurable and unpleasurable feelings. Then, of course, there's masturbating.

Learning how to masturbate? Start here

Sexologist Shamyra Howard, LCSW, lays down the essentials of self-pleasure:

1. Foreplay matters. Try picturing a scene that turns you on, and get your blood pumping by massaging your scalp or touching your breasts first.

2. When you feel warmed up, with clean hands, cup your mons, the area with hair above your labia.

3. With your hand in that position, press your fingers into your vulva and labia. Try moving your middle finger up and down, from your clitoris to your vaginal opening. This should increase lubrication; you can also use a couple drops of lube.

4. From there, use three or four fingers to "play the piano" on your clitoris, pressing each finger like a piano key in a wave motion. One after the other, lather, rinse, repeat!

5. If that's not working, try the "DJ" method, where you use your ring and middle finger to put light or medium pressure on your clitoris, and move it around like a DJ spinning a record. Try moving it back and forth, or in a circle.

6. Don't forget about rhythm. (This applies to vibrators, too!) Instead of trying a bunch of different techniques quickly, stick with one at a set pace to really find out if it's working for you.

Learning to Be Porn Literate

While it might seem counterintuitive, there's a lot you can learn about your own body and pleasure from porn, but that comes with caveats. And although there's no "wrong" type of porn to be interested in, sex educator and therapist Lexx Brown-James, PhD, advises looking for feminist-made porn as a jumping-off point. What does that look like? Brown-James says to look for porn that depicts and includes:

- Consent and consent negotiations
- Various shapes of bodies
- Various shapes of vulvas
- People of varied races and ethnicities
- Queer-presenting individuals
- Various sexual behaviors

Brown-James explains that it's important to see porn that accurately represents what America really looks like. Plus, she adds, it can be incredibly validating to see bodies like your own giving and receiving pleasure. The problem, of course, with mainstream porn that doesn't depict the above criteria is that it creates a really narrow view of what pleasure is and how it's supposed to be performed. If you only see white women with thin-lipped vulvas having sex with white men with gigantic penises, punched in with extreme closeups that hyperfocus on the genitals and nothing else . . . well, that's what pleasure will look like to you. It closes doors to so many different types of people, orientations, activities, and more that you will end up limiting and damaging your experience. If you see the same types of sex—a man pumping away inside a woman's vagina with no care paid to any other body parts—you might think there's something wrong with you if those methods, shockingly, don't do it for ya. Likewise, men who see those acts and only those may be more likely to repeat them with others. Meanwhile, feminist porn has the power to make all bodies feel desirable, and by offering a diverse array of activities, can give you inspiration for other things you might like to try. Solo masturbation videos can be especially educational if you're just starting out. Try searching for feminist porn roundups from well-trusted brands and websites (such as *Cosmo* or *Teen Vogue*), because they'll often give a short description of each site if you need more guidance.

TALKING TO YOUR PARTNER 301

It Starts in Your Mind

Now that you've figured out what you like on your own, how do you go about expressing that to a partner? For the purposes of this chapter, we're assuming that any hypothetical encounter is fully consensual, and that your partner is ready to hear feedback from you in good faith. If they are not, there are no tips in the world to fix the situation; they are simply not someone worthy of having sex with, full stop. So what can you do to communicate about what you want?

The first step is an attitude adjustment. If you find yourself generally keeping the volume down because you're worried being vocal in bed would be awkward, or would ruffle your partner's feathers, you can work to actively reframe your thinking. Justine Ang Fonte explains that in her eyes, there are three main reasons for sex. One is power, which is typically associated with assault; two is procreation, or trying to have a baby; and three is pleasure, or feeling good. If you're not using sex to feel powerful over someone else (which, again, bad), and you're not trying to conceive, your sole reason for sex is pleasure. So shouldn't you be maximizing every single moment? This isn't to say that sex can't also have the benefit of teaching you about yourself and bringing you closer to another person, but those are more like added bonuses: They're not the entire goal of having sex in that moment. The goal is to get pleasure from that encounter, and to give it, too. From there, it becomes easier to shift your thinking from *I'm not loving this, I guess I can just wait until it's over*, to *Why would I waste my time settling for sex that isn't making me feel good?* Sex without pleasure is like brushing your teeth without toothpaste. Why bother going through the motions if you're not getting what you came for?

Another attitude shift, as Brown-James explains, is to stop thinking about love and sex in terms of scarcity, and start thinking about them in terms of abundance. There exists a fear that if you've found someone who seems halfway decent, you don't want to do anything to "scare them off," because who knows when you'll meet someone else again? That's thinking about the world in terms of scarcity, and it's anxiety and fear talking. But you didn't get that idea out of thin air. Megahit shows like *Sex and the City* popularize myths like that one when Charlotte posits that you only get two great loves in your life. Two?! What if, instead of binding yourself to rigid rules about how many shots at a soulmate you get, you embraced the joy in knowing there are billions of people on the planet, and that love, lust, and attraction aren't finite commodities? You have so many chances. That's how you can shift to a mindset of abundance. The danger in sticking with the former is plain. Suppose you're sleeping with someone who doesn't make you feel entitled to speaking up. Brown-James asks, "If they won't act right in the bedroom, what else would they not be willing to compromise with you on? If it's showing up sexually, where else is it showing up, and is that going to be great for you?"

What to Say and Do First

Good sex doesn't necessarily mean having an orgasm. While I agree that if you're capable of orgasming (which not everyone is!) you should endeavor to explain those steps to someone else, a climax isn't the be-all and end-all of sex. Orgasms can be mysterious, tricky, and elusive! What worked to get you off yesterday might not do it today. You haven't failed if you don't come. The more important thing to focus on is having sex that feels good, which is a lot easier to achieve than a 100 percent orgasm occurrence rate.

1. Write it down

One way to build your confidence in your own communication skills is to practice writing down all the things that give you pleasure, and then the steps you'd take to stimulate those areas. Essentially, the same way you'd give someone directions to get to your house if they didn't know the area. What might start to feel second nature to you won't be obvious to a partner, so take the active step of writing down those cues with directions. This will help you recall them more naturally with a partner. It's one of the same theories behind taking notes or making flashcards for a test!

2. Talk with your clothes on

Next, it's important to have conversations about what your body likes *before* the sexy things are going down. If this is a longer-term courtship in the making, you'd likely have more time to build in these questions. Brown-James recommends asking things like, "I really want to see you naked. What's the best way to turn you on?" or "What do you like? What are your fantasies?" Starting with a question can be an easier way to open up a dialogue than blurting out a laundry list of things you want them to try—which isn't to say you shouldn't disclose those things! It might flow more naturally to ask first, have them ask you back in return, and then share.

3. Make communication a turn-on

With a one-night stand, your timing might be more limited, but you can still have a pre-sex conversation. Find a moment when you're still fully or mostly clothed, like when you're waiting outside for the Uber to take you both back to campus, and say, "I can't wait to get you home, what's the first thing we should do together?" between make-out sessions. From there, it's easy to drop in, "Mmmm, yes please, I also want you to [insert sex thing here]." The purpose of these conversations is simple: Now you've both laid a groundwork of how to make sex good for you, and that's starting with a leg up—and maybe some other parts, too.

It's crucial to share things you like beforehand—and equally things that are off the table for you. Leah, eighteen, who attends college in North Carolina, told me about the night she went home with a guy after hanging out at a frat party. Leah will typically share if something feels good in the moment, but she admits that there's not usually a lot of conversation surrounding pleasure before she gets intimate with a guy. "We don't have a business meeting before everything goes down," she quips. When, out of nowhere, he slapped her across the face when they were having sex, she knew right away that wasn't something she liked. But Leah didn't say as much to that guy. Not in the moment, not afterward, and not when she slept with him again sometime later. She told me that she would have brought it up if he did it a second time, but since he didn't, she decided to let it go. When I ask why the hesitancy, Leah explains, "I didn't want it to be uncomfortable and I also didn't want him to feel some type of way. I guess he should, because he did it. But I didn't want any of that. I just didn't want to get into it." Part of me gets it. Even though this was behavior she clearly didn't like, that shocked her in a bad way, Leah acknowledged it didn't physically hurt her. This is what I mean when I say we're collectively lowering the bar and not putting our own pleasure first. We accept things that rub us the wrong way because we don't want to come face-to-face with a conversation that has the potential to be uncomfortable. To be clear, her partner was the one in the wrong. You should never introduce rough sex activities without getting your partner's consent first. And while I understand that speaking up in the moment or even after isn't always easy, and sometimes might even be dangerous if you suspect your partner could get violent, but if you feel it's safe to do so, please try. Maybe this guy was just an idiot who thought all women liked that. Maybe he had an ex who loved it.

⚠️ **By not letting someone know when a boundary is crossed, you're potentially reinforcing behavior that could get their next partner hurt. Speaking up for your own pleasure is a radical act.**

In-the-Moment Pleasure Instruction

Okay, so you've met someone great! You know what you like! Maybe you've even talked a little about the things that turn you on . . . or, maybe you haven't. If not, there's hope! You still have in-the-moment communication tactics to help you and your partner have a pleasurable experience. What does that look like? Brown-James explains it's all about feedback and direction. Saying things like, "Mmm I like that. Can you do that over here? Take it a little bit deeper. I really love it when you slow down. I really love it when you touch me here, or kiss me there, or bite me there." That direction can be incredibly hot, turning your partner on and making it easier for them to make you feel good in the process. Perhaps most important, she adds, it prevents them from "fumbling and bumbling around and trying to figure you out like a puzzle."

You can also try "masturbation shows," where you both masturbate in front of each other to better exhibit the movements and touches you like.

You can play with this concept in lots of different ways. Maybe you want to lie close to each other on a bed and masturbate at the same time. Maybe you want to take turns watching each other. Maybe, as Brown-James suggests, you want to make a game of it and let your partner "hide" and watch you from somewhere out of sight for a voyeuristic turn-on. Then there's physically manipulating your partner's hand to show them the motions in a more direct way. This is also great for partners of different abilities, like those who are nonverbal or hearing impaired.

Finally, don't make "sex directions" the only thing you talk about during sex. Byers notes that if you cultivate a sex life that's full of ongoing verbal communication, it won't feel so daunting when you need to speak up about what's not working for you. Tell them their ass looks incredible in that underwear, say how good something feels when it does, talk about how you've been thinking about doing this all day, even the weather, it doesn't matter! It's all about creating an environment where feedback is welcomed, not feared. We can't let a fear of ruining the mood ruin the sex instead. It's the compliment sandwich of dirty talk—name some things you love, some things you want to work on, and more things you love. As Sandra Byers says, "Silent sex is bad sex; we should be talking all the time."

So You've Been Faking It . . .

A lot of us have been there. One study of college students shows that 50 percent of women (and 25 percent of men) have faked an orgasm, be it during intercourse, oral sex, or even phone sex.[2] The study goes on to note that some of the main reasons people report faking an orgasm are wanting the sex to end, not wanting to hurt their partner's feelings, or because they didn't think they were going to orgasm anyway. But when you fake an orgasm, you're depriving your partner of a chance to genuinely make you feel amazing, and you're sending a clear message that what they're doing works for you, when in fact it may not be.

If you think it doesn't matter for hookups and one-night stands, you're wrong. Even if you never intend to see this person again, you're sending them out into the world with a false belief that they're an orgasm-inducing god and reinforcing the belief to *yourself* that you don't really deserve sex that feels good. What if you thought it was just a fling but decide later on it could be more serious? Then you're stuck explaining why something that they thought felt amazing for you before only elicits a flatline response from you now. Plus, furthering the belief that an orgasm is just so integral to sex that we need to fake it if it doesn't happen erodes the idea that good sex can exist without a climax. We need to normalize telling our partners that we love the way they made us feel, with or without our muscles contracting in an orgasm-specific pattern! Being honest about sex from the get-go helps more than you might think. As with everything with sex, this comes with a caveat. If you're in a situation where you feel unsafe, and you believe faking an orgasm will end a potentially dangerous sexual encounter so you can leave, do so. Don't think twice.

You're not a bad person if you've faked an orgasm, neither are you a bad feminist nor a bad partner. But if you find yourself wondering why you can't just let out a few half-hearted moans to stroke some guy's ego, try channeling the energy of Adelaide, a senior at a large university in upstate New York. Adelaide has always felt entitled to speak up for herself during sex, in part because her early relationships were with partners who modeled communication surprisingly well for teenage straight guys. They asked her what she liked, how things were working for her, and shared what they liked with her, too. Because her first sexual encounters were in the context of ongoing relationships with plenty of chances to talk, she developed that same sense of communication-as-the-default, too. That goes doubly for orgasm-faking. When the topic comes up, she blurts out, "I was hoping you were going to ask this question! This is my favorite story to tell." When Adelaide was eighteen, she vividly recalls seeing a tweet that said something along the lines of "Why would you fake an orgasm? Let him know that his dick game is weak." This is obviously oversimplified—you can have great "dick game" even if your partner doesn't climax! But there's truth in that. What's really gained by letting someone believe a lie? Adelaide identified with the message immediately. "I held it with me ever since," she explains. "If they're not getting me off, they shouldn't receive the satisfaction that they are because it doesn't benefit either of us. They're gonna think that they have done something when they haven't." So when it comes to sex, she applies this theory in a straightforward but thoughtful way. If she can tell an orgasm is just not in the cards, Adelaide will tell her partner—sooner rather than later. She's found that letting sex drag on for longer than it's pleasurable just heightens frustration for everyone. She keeps things light and nonjudgmental by saying, "Hey, this feels really good, but I don't think it's gonna happen for me tonight." From there, she'll either suggest they give it a break for a bit or try something else (think: mutual masturbation, massage, etc.) before they end the night with some talking.

If you do find yourself in a situation where you've been letting your partner believe you've orgasmed on an ongoing basis, and you want to set the record straight, you've got options. Brown-James, who's worked with couples who've been together for years and are only now starting to address this issue, says for the partner that's been misled, it can feel like a serious betrayal. If you've already gone down that path but want to course correct, she doesn't necessarily recommend coming in hot with a tearful admission that you've been lying all this time. Instead, try couching the conversation in terms of exploration, so you can introduce behaviors you do enjoy. Like, "Hey there's this thing I've really wanted to try. Would you be down to hear about it?" Getting your partner on board to talk about it can start you both from a place of a willingness to learn. And if they keep asking about or trying things that don't do it for you? A simple, "Eh, that hasn't been working for me as much lately. What else can we try?" can redirect without causing hurt feelings.

℮℮℮℮

Thinking so deeply about pleasure has me considering the times when I felt the least of it. I remember dutifully moaning through sex with guys whose only goal seemed to be shaking the headboard in an ever faster rhythm. I watched, quizzically, as they spit on (both of!!) our junk, thinking it was a perfect substitute for lube. Less egregious on their part, I faked orgasm after orgasm if I felt like we even approached "this is tolerable" territory. I would have encouraged anything that even had *potential* to feel good. My bar was on the ground.

Then I started dating more seriously. I remember, somewhere around my mid-twenties, meeting a guy I liked a lot. I knew things would never work out if our entire sexual history was built upon, if not outright lies, stretching the truth. More important, I didn't want to be with someone I couldn't trust to handle my honesty without seeing it as an affront to their masculinity. So I came clean about our first few nights together. Namely, that I hadn't always asked for what I needed to make the experience as good as I had implied it had been. Maybe I didn't need to, maybe I did it without the tact I've offered in this chapter, but I did it. It was uncomfortable and hurt someone I care about deeply, but I needed to value my pleasure as much as I did someone else's if I wanted to make a life with them. And now I use a vibrator whenever I feel like it! And now you know it, too. Maybe it's a cringey overshare the world didn't need (probably), but if it makes you feel even the tiniest bit better about asking for what you want, I'm glad to have set the record straight.

6.

Queer in College

Social Life and Sex on Campus

I don't have a fun/funny/embarrassing/horrifying story from my misguided-ish youth this time around. This chapter is all about the queer college experience, and as a cisgender straight woman, I don't have much—if any—personal insight to add. Sure, I could go on about how I used to make out with my straight girlfriends at parties for the amusement of any guy watching. I now know that this encourages harassment of actual queer women from ignorant people. We'll talk more about allyship later in this chapter, but a big tenet of supporting a group that you don't belong to is getting out of the way and letting them speak for themselves. So without further ado, much less me, much more everyone else.

ℓℓℓℓ

You've probably heard some of the frightening and grim statistics when it comes to queer youth. Just 24 percent feel like they can fully be themselves at home with their family.[1] Queer youth are almost three times as likely to seriously consider suicide, compared to their straight peers.[2] And it's especially important to acknowledge the burdens in addition to homophobia faced by queer youth of color, 80 percent of whom have personally experienced racism.[3] Gender identity matters, too: 24 percent of trans students have been threatened or hurt with a weapon at school, compared to just 6 percent of cisgender males and 4 percent of cisgender females.[4] The struggles LGBTQ youth face both at home and in school are palpable, but there is also very real joy, optimism, and freedom.

LGBTQ VOCAB 101

A Handy Glossary

Before we dive deeper, if you've ever felt a little lost or confused when it comes to LGBTQ terminology, you are not the only one. And that's fine! Even if you had excellent and inclusive sex ed, you might forget some of these terms, or occasionally use them incorrectly. That's okay, too; everyone has to start somewhere. That's how you learn. Adapted from the GLAAD Media Reference Guide, here are some key terms about sexual orientation, gender identity, and queer community you should know.

ASEXUAL

An adjective used to describe people who do not experience sexual attraction. A person can also be aromantic, meaning they do not experience romantic attraction. Some asexual people may describe themselves as "ace."

BIOLOGICAL SEX

The classification of a person as male or female. At birth, infants are assigned a sex, usually based on the appearance of their external anatomy. (This is what is written on the birth certificate.) A person's sex, however, is actually a combination of bodily characteristics including: chromosomes, hormones, internal and external reproductive organs, and secondary sex characteristics.

BISEXUAL, BI

A person who has the capacity to form enduring physical, romantic, and/or emotional attractions to those of the same gender or to those of another gender. People may experience this attraction in differing ways and degrees over their lifetime. Bisexual people need not have had specific sexual experiences to be bisexual; in fact, they need not have had any sexual experience at all to identify as bisexual.

CISGENDER

A term used by some to describe people whose gender identity aligns with the sex they were assigned at birth. "Cis-" is a Latin prefix meaning "on the same side as," and is therefore an antonym of "trans-."

GAY

The adjective used to describe people whose enduring physical, romantic, and/or emotional attractions are to people of the same sex. Sometimes lesbian is the preferred term for women.

GENDER EXPRESSION

External manifestations of gender, expressed through a person's name, pronouns, clothing, haircut, behavior, voice, and/or body characteristics. Society identifies these cues as masculine and feminine, although what is considered masculine or feminine changes over time and varies by culture. Typically, people seek to align their gender expression with their gender identity, rather than the sex they were assigned at birth.

GENDER IDENTITY

A person's internal, deeply held sense of their gender. Most people understand gender as a binary of either male or female. For many people, their gender identity does not fit neatly into one of those two choices (*see* non-binary and/or genderqueer). Unlike gender expression, gender identity is not visible to others.
See also cisgender and transgender

GENDER NON-CONFORMING

A term used to describe some people whose gender expression is different from conventional expectations of masculinity and femininity. While many gender non-conforming people identify as transgender, not all of them do. Many people have gender expressions that are not entirely conventional.

HETEROSEXUAL

An adjective used to describe people whose enduring physical, romantic, and/or emotional attraction is to people of the opposite sex. Also *straight*.

INTERSEX

A term describing people born with reproductive or sexual anatomy and/or a chromosome pattern that can't be classified as typically male or female. Those variations are also sometimes referred to as differences of sex development (DSD). Avoid the outdated and derogatory term "hermaphrodite." While some people can have an intersex condition and also identify as transgender, the two are separate and should not be conflated.

NON-BINARY

Terms used by some people who experience their gender identity and/or gender expression as falling outside the categories of man and woman. They may define their gender as falling somewhere in between man and woman, or they may define it as wholly different from these terms. Some may also use the term "gender fluid." Many non-binary people prefer gender-neutral pronouns, which may include they/them, xe, ze, sie, and others, or a combination.

QUEER

An adjective used by some people whose sexual orientation is not exclusively heterosexual. Typically, for those who identify as queer, the terms lesbian, gay, and bisexual are perceived to be too limiting and/or fraught with cultural connotations they feel don't apply to them. Some people may use queer, or more commonly genderqueer, to describe their gender identity and/or gender expression. Once considered a pejorative term, queer has been reclaimed by some LGBTQ people to describe themselves; however, it is not a universally accepted term even within the LGBTQ community.

SEXUAL ORIENTATION

A person's enduring physical, romantic, and/or emotional attraction to another person. Gender identity and sexual orientation are not the same. Regardless of your gender identity, your sexual orientation may be straight, lesbian, gay, bisexual, or queer.

TRANSGENDER

An umbrella term for people whose gender identity and/or gender expression differs from the sex they were assigned at birth. People under the transgender umbrella may describe themselves using one or more of a wide variety of terms—including transgender. Some of those terms are defined in this glossary. Use the descriptive term preferred by the person. Many transgender people seek medical treatment to bring their bodies into alignment with their gender identity, which may include hormone replacement therapy, surgery, both, or neither. But not all transgender people can or will take those steps, and being transgender is not dependent upon physical appearance or medical procedures.

Reframing Unique Dilemmas

Some of the quandaries LGBTQ people in college face may be the exact same as their straight peers, and others may be more nuanced hurdles and triumphs specific to the queer experience. Take Eloise, a recent grad from an art school in the Northeast, who primarily dates other women. When I asked her what her chief concerns were when it comes to the dating scene in college, she started with the basics. Sometimes just finding people who are interested in you is a challenge in and of itself: She describes the double complication of figuring out if someone is queer and then on top of that, if they're into her. (Given that straight people are the majority demographic-wise, they only have to contend with the latter.) Eloise explains that there's no monolithic approach to queer courtship: Some queer people can feel confident initiating a romantic connection in any space, some just in queer spaces like clubs and gay bars, and some perhaps only on dating apps. But even the apps,

Eloise explains, have their pitfalls. She once matched with a girl who she knew was queer, because it said so on all her socials. Then after going on what she thought was a date, she stopped to ask if things were romantic or platonic between them, to which the other woman replied, "Oh, I thought we were just hanging out." Eloise recalls the hurtful mixup, saying, "Queer people also just want queer friends." Granted, I think the onus was more on Eloise's "date" to be upfront about what she was looking for, but it does illustrate a difference between queer and straight experiences. The assumption, however unfair and limiting, is that if a man met a woman on an app and asked her to get a coffee with him, she'd probably correctly assume it was a date, given the odds that they're both straight and that men and women don't often pursue friendship via apps. "I've fantasized in the past, like 'Oh if the roles were different here, if the situation was different, I would just like, *know*, and I wouldn't have to ask her.' I wouldn't have to make a move and see how they react," Eloise tells me.

Then there are the microaggressions, many of which can feel very macro in the moment. I've heard stories of queer women on dates at bars, where straight guys will approach and try to pick them up, either not believing they're there together, or harassing them to make out. Eloise recalled a similar incident, when two men wouldn't stop bothering her and her date on a park bench, and she had to adopt a hypermasculine persona to get them to scram. She wonders if it would have been necessary if they had been a straight couple.

I also spoke with Mirai, a senior at a large private university, who is bisexual. She hasn't had many romantic encounters with women, she explains, partly because she feels like she doesn't know how to approach them. She's seen models for heterosexual dating from TV and straight friends, but less so when it comes to pursuing women. "There are some friends I can talk to sometimes, but I don't have a lot of gay friends who have a lot of experience. So it's hard to be like, 'help me!'" she explains.

This, added to some homophobic experiences she's endured, makes it more daunting to explore that part of her identity. Mirai has met women who have outright told her, "Don't hit on me if you're queer." She also recalls attending a summer program on the campus of another university. She met a girl there who was queer who told her about an awful situation with her roommate. At the start of the program the pair had no trouble feeling comfortable in their dorm; they'd walk around in their underwear without thinking twice. Then when the roommate found out Mirai's friend was queer, all of a sudden she started changing in the bathroom and acted much more conservative around her. This type of ignorance fuels untrue stereotypes: No, gay people are not trolling their dorms trying to hit on every straight person they see just because they have the type of genitalia they're most often attracted to. It doesn't work like that. And any belief to the contrary can create toxic environments, preventing queer people from being themselves.

I'll be upfront that this chapter can't offer a far-reaching solution to end homophobia in college, or anyplace else for that matter. Education and exposure help, but not everyone wants to learn. What I can do is offer practical tips and new ways of thinking about old problems to help queer students pursue happier and healthier relationships. I told you there'd be optimism and joy in this chapter, and here it is.

Shannon Sennott, a sex therapist who teaches at Smith College School of Social Work, describes a major shift among queer youth today that gives her immense hope. In both her students and patients, she's witnessed a group of young adults who feel entitled to what they deserve in their relationships: affirming, positive connection. "I get a lot of college-age, queer people who are designated female, who definitely feel like their sexual identity and their sexual practices are one hundred percent founded in a consent-based model. That is just so different than any other age category that I have seen in my practice over the last fifteen years," Sennott explains. "I think, in a way, it sort of puts them in a place of empowerment." That empowerment can breed confidence for queer people to carve out the space they need to truly understand their sexual orientation, and license to identify in whatever way fits. Part of that is the advent of the internet opening up young adults to tons of information about queer identity and terminology. Let's say you've spent your adolescence wondering why you're not all that interested in sex with anyone, you might feel alone or out of place.

Meeting others who have had similar experiences can be life-affirming.

Then, you read online about what it means to be asexual, and you connect with other people who identify with the term on forums and message boards, and suddenly your whole world expands. Meeting others who have had similar experiences can be life-affirming. While it's important not to put everyone in a box and assume there can't be more to them than the identifying labels they use, there can be so much power in claiming your identity with terms that feel right to you. "Once we have a label, people can come together and rise up around it," Sennott says.

This type of confidence and fair sense of entitlement can help us see the upshot in scenarios we once thought of as problems. When it comes to the "Who the hell are the other queer people around here and are they into me?" debacle, Sennott assures that it is a really normal and relatable issue. Instead of shifting to the "If I were straight this would be easier" mindset, she suggests first exploring whether or not the model of heterosexuality you're looking at is even healthy in the first place. The assumption that straight people often operate under, that anybody of the opposite sex is fair game to be eagerly pursued, is damaging for a lot of reasons. For one, it diminishes the safety of women pursuing friendships with straight men, since the default assumption would likely be, "Oh, she's into me. Must pursue accordingly or rebuff entirely." Plus, a fear of "leading a guy on" probably stops a lot of women from even trying in the first place. It also assumes that we can look at a person and just magically read their mind about who they are what they want: That's a man, I'm a woman, we'll hook up and have vaginal intercourse, the end. As Sennott points out, that cuts us off from having to develop the language to learn about potential partners and their intimate needs. Queer people, likely out of necessity, tend to develop more nuanced ways to get and give this information because there's less of that unhealthy assumption going on. Not every woman is going to be available and into you. There's no one type of sex assumed to be the "default." As a result, you need to learn how to ask questions to get those answers. Isn't it a gift to be able to talk freely about intimacy with your potential partners? (Thankfully, we've talked a lot about how to ask for what you need and want in this book, so you get to be an expert!) A quick tip from Sennott for finding queer partners on dating apps: Use as many descriptive identity labels as you're comfortable with (queer, nonbinary, bisexual, poly, etc.). It's a form of activism in and of itself because it can normalize these terms for people who are unfamiliar with them, but the benefit for you is that it can draw in like-minded people more easily. Plus, Sennott adds, someone who may have skipped over you otherwise could be enticed by one sliver of shared identity, and a spark might ignite where it wouldn't have otherwise.

Another concern brought up by students I interviewed is the notion that the queer college dating scene is incestuous. No, not literally! (And not my words, either.) But the reality is there are likely more straight people on your campus than queer people. It's just math! So there's bound to be a bit of overlap between who's dated whom. It can start to feel like everyone in your friend group has been with everyone else, creating this image of a family who fucks. (I'm sorry!) If your school is in a big city, you may have more luck expanding your dating pool, but on smaller campuses it may just be a hurdle you learn to love over the next four years. Sennott suggests thinking about it as a gift rather than a burden. Dipping your toes into dating as an out queer person can be super overwhelming at first, so wouldn't it be a good thing if some of your first encounters were with someone you know well, someone who's been vetted by your friend group? It also gives you a chance to talk more about openness with your friends. Straight women are often socialized to be very secretive about sex, to "claim" a guy if they've slept with him and make him off-limits to friends forever. Queer people don't always have that luxury given the smaller dating pool, so it forces useful conversations with friends about where those boundaries are. What they're comfortable seeing, what they want you to know about how they're feeling, etc. Plus, wouldn't it be kind of cool to know your potential partner's dating résumé from word of mouth before you hook up? If I knew in advance who sucked at giving head and who didn't, I could have saved myself from a lot of thoroughly average sex. Sennott, of course, diplomatically interjects: "And if you really like them, now you know, and you can teach them that!"

Sometimes, however, the key to healthier relationships with yourself and others is time. Rosalie, twenty-one, just finished her junior year at a historically women's college. Rosalie is trans, and was surprised that even though there are other trans students attending her school, she couldn't find any other transfeminine students on her campus when she arrived as a freshman. She's built a strong community of friends over the years, and while she doesn't feel isolated per se, in her words she does occasionally get that pang of "Oh right, some of my experiences will just never be shared by any of the people on this campus." She initially wanted to get in touch with other trans women at her school to build connection, get the lay of the land, and find out about their experiences. It was a bit of a letdown when it didn't happen. Even without a community of trans women, Rosalie loves the sense of safety and openness she's felt from the student body. She especially appreciates that professors and students alike always make it a point to request people's pronouns, and many will use the singular they/them to refer to someone whose pronouns they don't know until they learn otherwise. This inclusive environment doesn't mean college has been without challenges. Using the bathrooms at a historically women's college has been a point of stress for her. Rosalie explains that she has a deep voice, which creates some anxiety for her in these spaces. "If no one saw my face as I was talking, and didn't know me or wasn't friends with me, I'm always worried, what if they're worried? What if I'm causing distress or fear for them?" she says. It's complicated by the fact that there's only one set of bathrooms per dorm, and students often have their cis boyfriends over to visit. "I just don't want to make anyone feel unsafe or concerned, but that's at the cost of me sitting there worrying if I say anything that might scare someone, which isn't the best mental thing to have." Over time, however, Rosalie has developed a new mindset that's helped her quiet some of those nagging voices. She tells herself, "This is the school that I'm going to. I belong here. I have gone here for three years now. This is a space where I'm meant to be and allowed to be. And the people around me—I just have to trust aren't going to be concerned that I exist there." It's a very powerful mantra to consider: You belong anywhere you are. Rosalie told me she learned there's going to be another transfeminine student

You belong anywhere you are.

joining her on campus next year, and she's thinking about reaching out. She's looking forward to being the person she wished she had found when she first started college.

How to Come Out about Anything

Coming out, the decision to share your sexual orientation or your gender identity with others, is personal. There's no schedule to go by or set script to use, but there are some groundwork-level principles you can use to speak your truth to others, courtesy of Shannon Sennott. Bonus: These tools work for everything from "Hey mom, I'm gay!" to "Wanna try a strap-on?" Tips for tough convos, right this way.

1. Find a supportive person for practice

People with marginalized or stigmatized identities can face a certain amount of internalized shame after a lifetime of getting the message that who they are or what they want is outside the norm. So finding someone to talk things through with, someone who you know won't shame you, is key. This is important for a couple of reasons. One, you'll learn how you want to say it and develop the muscle memory of having done it already. Just about anything is easier and less scary the second time around! Second, you'll have the experience of getting a kind, affirming response from whoever you chose to talk to. And if you don't have anyone in your circle who fits the bill, or even if you're just not ready, you can get some of the same benefits by simply writing it down as if you were going to share it with someone. Read it aloud, make edits, practice it looking in a mirror, whatever helps. Feeling ownership of the words you want to say is key to having the confidence to deliver them. Give yourself an affirming smile or pat on the back when you're done— you deserve it!

2. Set up your audience to have a positive experience

It's important that you get the buy-in from whoever you're sharing with. Even telling your partner something intimate, like wanting to experiment with kink or BDSM for the first time, can feel super terrifying to ask for, but don't forget your audience might be coming to the convo with their own baggage. Make sure you ask first, giving them a bit of a preview of what the conversation will be like. Sennott suggests trying, "I have something I'd like to share. It's about a sexual practice that I'm interested in. I was hoping that we could talk more about it, would you be open to doing that?" If they say no, your best bet is to find someone else. If they're not ready or able to hear what you have to say, the experience won't be positive for you either. And if you're nervous, it can be really helpful to say so. Try, "This is something that I've realized about myself and am excited to explore. But I feel nervous to share this because I've never told anybody. I'm hopeful that you'll be able to hear this because you've always been so supportive." This sets your friend up to know just how much you value them, which will prime them to be extra kind and affirming.

3. Timing is everything

Whether you're telling your "preview partner" or the ultimate intended audience, be deliberate about where and when you have these conversations so that you can have a clear head. You'll want to do it when neither of you is hungry, and you're both totally sober. Hunger can be a distracting and aggravating emotion, and I don't think I need to explain to you, my very smart and discerning reader, why you shouldn't have important conversations while smashed. Then there's the literal time, which is daytime! In the evening you're more likely to be exhausted from the day and not fully present, or to have already been drinking. Plus, many people's anxieties ramp up at night, so best to avoid it. Sennott suggests a substance-free daytime picnic to check all these boxes. Planning the timing matters not only for the reasons above, but because keeping it all pent up and blurting it out at the wrong moment can be actively harmful. You might say something that's not exactly what you meant, or your intended audience might be taken by surprise and not able to offer you the support you deserve. So plan ahead; you'll be glad you did!

There's a lot about coming out that's up to you, and if it feels like the right supportive environment at 5:01 PM, just when the sun is starting to set and you're getting ready for dinner, don't let that stop you. These aren't unforgiving rules and no one is grading your exam, but hopefully this can be a good starting point to start sharing more of yourself with your partners, friends, and family.

An Unexpected Gift: Queer Sex as Liberation

I've done my best to write this book so that the sex stuff—learning about what brings you pleasure, asking for what you want, talking intimacy with partners, navigating consent—works for any two bodies (or three! Or four!) who are having the aforementioned sex. But in discussing some of the differences queer people might experience when it comes to their sex lives, one uplifting topic came to light. These encounters can be liberating in ways not all straight people can or will experience.

To back things up a bit, what does liberation in this sense mean? Liberation, Sennott explains, is connected to the idea of making progress or being affirmed by others. It's not often something that can happen on its own in a bubble. "These experiences have to be met with a certain level of radical, inclusive acceptance by other people. It feeds itself. [Liberation] is a network community experience," she adds.

Queer sex may present an opportunity to call your own shots. Think of it like this: When a cis straight man and a cis straight woman get together with the intent of having sex, it's likely they both think of the culmination of that sex as PIV intercourse. That's the end game. Sure, there may be some oral-sex-as-foreplay thrown in, but the "ultimate" goal is usually the same. What might you do if you didn't have that goal? What other body parts might you explore? What questions might you ask your partner, what might you learn about each other? How might that change the focus to what feels the best, not just what you think you're supposed to do? It's not just about an absence of penises in the mix, either. Lots of queer people, including women, may have penises, but that doesn't mean vaginal penetration via said penis is going to be part of the sexual experience for them at all. Some may prefer using a strap-on. Some may feel like vaginal penetration is heteronormative and therefore misogynistic. Some may experience gender dysphoria if they use their penis during sex. The point being, freeing yourself from what sex is supposed to be can open new and more pleasurable doors. And perhaps there's something to that: After all, 62 percent of straight women report having orgasms during sex, compared to a whopping nearly 75 percent of gay women.[5] And think about this: As many as 21 percent of women experience sexual pain during intercourse,[6] and yet something that hurts 1 out of 5 women is still considered to be the default form of straight sex. In this way, Sennott adds, perhaps more straight women could take a page out of the book of queer sex.

QUEER COMMUNITY 101

The Good, the Bad, and the Messy

There is a notion that once a queer person can escape the confines of a rejecting family away at college and find their queer community that every other obstacle is out of the way. Mercifully, this may be true for a lot of people, but not everyone. Faith, a junior at an HBCU (historically Black colleges and universities) in the Mid-Atlantic, has experienced a bit of both. Faith, who uses both she/her and they/them pronouns, is a lesbian who describes themself as masculine-presenting, identifying with the term "stud." They grew up with a family whose Nigerian culture and Christian values weren't always aligned with how they wanted to present. "My family thinks you're going to get pneumonia in your knee if you wear ripped jeans," they quip. Faith's grandma expected them to be wearing heels and skirts all the time at college, a missive Faith is thrilled to get to ignore. Faith knows that gender identity and gender expression are two different things, and it brings them joy to switch up their looks and find what feels right. "I love that when you're in college, you can find yourself. You can explore as much as you want. Honestly, college is a trial and error, and I love that, because I'm not home getting nagged with someone telling me in one ear to do something, and someone not," Faith explains. "If you're trying to find out what you want to be and what you are, you're in a place to do it. And you can easily find people who are like you."

But that doesn't mean all of their experiences with the queer community have been perfect. An important cause for them is bringing light to the discrimination masculine-presenting Black and Brown queer people face. Just because they dress masculine and embrace hard edges of style doesn't mean they aren't still soft at times. It doesn't mean they don't like getting their hair or nails done occasionally. But some of Faith's past partners have wanted to put them in a box and keep them there. Faith has noticed colorism plays a role here, too: Darker-skinned Black queer people are also unfairly portrayed as more aggressive. Faith recalls one girl she dated who expected them to act masculine and dominant all the time, because it fit her idea of how Faith's outsides should match their insides. Faith explained it turned their girlfriend on when they'd act macho, so she'd pick fights trying to bring out the aggro energy. So her girlfriend would taunt her, posting on Instagram posing with other girls alongside cutesy captions. When Faith didn't take the bait and instead wanted to talk about it rationally, she'd be dismissive. To have so much of themself erased and to be boiled down to just one element of how they present was hurtful and disappointing to Faith, to say the least. "There's so much pressure, because if I dress or act mascu- line, people will be like, 'Okay, well she wants to be the man.' And then if I dress feminine, they're like, 'What type of stud are you even anyway?' It's like you can't win."

I spoke to Sabra L. Katz-Wise, PhD, an assistant professor at Boston Children's Hospital with joint appointments at Harvard Medical School and the Harvard T. H. Chan School of Public Health. Her work focuses on LGBTQ people's identity development and health inequities and so she gets what Faith is going through. Katz-Wise looks at where the sys- tem fails queer youth. She explains, for example, that sexual minority women actually have a higher risk of teen pregnancy, likely due to lack of counseling from healthcare providers who incorrectly assume they aren't at risk for pregnancy. But a bisexual woman may have intercourse with men, a lesbian may date a woman who has a penis, and so on. It's just one way health institutions can leave queer youth behind. Like oth- ers I've spoken to, Katz-Wise doesn't just see a grim picture of inequity. She sees a community that's vastly creative and vigorously engaged in activism that serves their communities. And she also sees finding your community or chosen family as critical to your overall well-being and protective of your mental health. Everyone deserves a wide circle of people who affirm and accept them unconditionally, but building your network is especially important for those who didn't have the most ac- cepting of families.

Even if you find a queer community, however, it doesn't mean you won't face the type of ignorance Faith did. Katz-Wise acknowledges that these stereotypes are prevalent and harmful, even within their own ranks. "I think part of this is really the need for our society to move beyond these very strict binary expectations around gender," she explains. She has hope that eventually Faith will find partners who accept them in all of their complexity, but their predicament might offer a moment for a bit of education. Noting that it is in no way someone's responsibility to educate in the face of ignorance, Katz-Wise suggests that it could feel powerful or comforting to assert yourself and say, "Hey, gender identity and gender expression are two different things, and how I choose to look is not all there is to who I am. I'm looking to be with someone who sees that." Beyond that specific scenario, we just have to make space for one another to be able to redefine ourselves as necessary. One of the biggest misconceptions Katz-Wise sees is the assumption that gender identity and sexual orientation are stable across time for everybody. You might identify your whole young adulthood as lesbian, and then perhaps you notice some shifts in your attractions and the term "bisexual" fits you better. She/her pronouns might feel right for a while, and they/them might ultimately ring even truer. The most important thing to keep in mind, according to Katz-Wise, is that this is all normal.

QUEER COMMUNITY 201
Building Your Chosen Family

By now you may be wondering, how do you build your community? It's important to acknowledge that straight people don't always struggle to find mentors in the way queer people might. After all, if straight girls have a question about sex or dating that their parents won't answer, they may have an older sister or aunt or care provider who knows exactly what they're going through. It's not guaranteed that queer youth have a queer relative immediately accessible to them.

There are pros and cons to searching out your crew. Katz-Wise bemoans the closure of many lesbian bars, which are great places to meet friends and partners alike. But, despite their decline in prevalence, not everyone finds them to be so useful. Faith, for example, notices that lesbian bars are full of straight friends tagging along with queer peers, or packed with women in relationships.

But another strategy to find mentors, make friends, or meet potential partners is to join community organizations. Does your campus have a queer peer-educator program? An activism outreach group? It seems obvious, but start with the basics of where you might find likewise-identified people. And if your school doesn't already have a queer club or association, Katz-Wise suggests starting with your own interests and forming a group yourself. Do you love writing? Why not start up a queer writing workshop? A photography club? You get the idea. This doesn't mean you're going to try to jump into the pants of anyone who's showing up at your club to work on their art, but it can be a start to putting down roots with people at school who will understand you and lift you up. And who knows, maybe your new writing buddy has a hot friend they will introduce you to later down the line!

ALLYSHIP 101

Allyship—being there, supporting, and lifting up others from a group of which you are not a member—is often thought of as performed by straight people to queer people. And while that's certainly a component, there's allyship that must take place within the queer community itself.

Here to help sort out how it's done is Sophia Arredondo, former director of Education and Youth Programs for GLSEN (which used to be called the Gay, Lesbian, and Straight Education Network). For her, allyship centers around three more A's: assumptions, affirming, and advocating.

1. Assumptions

So much of what we get wrong about allyship stems from our assumptions. Too often we assume someone's gender identity and the pronouns they use just by looking at their outward expression like clothes, accessories, hair, and mannerisms, but it's critical not to assume that someone's gender identity, sexual orientation, or use of pronouns is based on their appearance. When you make these snap judgments, you don't allow that person to feel fully seen or accepted for who they are, and you erase and invalidate them. It also prevents you from making what could be true meaningful connections, which can't happen unless someone is being their whole self with you.

Even well-meaning allies slip up, but that erasure can have real consequences. Take, for example, the phenomenon of bisexual erasure. "I think a lot of bi folks feel erased in a community that is supposed to be their own," Arredondo explains. The passing comments like, "Oh, that person is only calling themself bi until they come out as gay" are incredibly hurtful. Alejandra, a senior who goes to school in Pennsylvania, has dealt with this firsthand. When she first came out as bisexual, she says, no one believed her. Then when she started a relationship with a woman, her mom just assumed she was a lesbian. It was all incredibly frustrating, especially because she felt grounded in the term "bisexual." "I'm not one way or another. Like, I literally am what I say I am. There's so little trust in college women about their sexuality," Alejandra says. These things add up and can threaten a person's self-esteem. (It's worth noting that some believe the term "bisexual" itself is too binary and erases attraction to people of other genders or nonbinary individuals, so some prefer the term "bi+" to account for attraction to others beyond the male/female binary.) "I've met many a queer woman who is married or dating a trans man and is read as a straight couple, and they also may have that feeling of erasure," Arredondo explains. If you just assume instead of getting to know and asking, you're telling them that you don't think their queer identity is real or valid. And we can all do better than that.

2. Affirming

Perhaps the opposite of assuming and ignoring is affirming, when you acknowledge that someone is exactly who they know themself to be without question, and offer your support. If you had a queer friend who came home and told you how upset they were to have been ignored by waitstaff on their romantic date because people assumed they weren't a couple, you can look them in the eye and tell them how much that sucks, but that you're here for them and you see them.

This is especially critical for trans youth. One of the easiest and most straightforward things you can do to affirm trans youth (or any trans person!) is to use their correct pronouns and the name they ask to be called. School roll calls can be fraught for trans people, because attendance rosters aren't always updated from the names students were assigned at birth. Fight for your school to have correct pronouns in their information system. And if necessary, remind your professors that it doesn't take a legal name change for them to update their own personal class rosters so they can affirm their students' identities.

What about pronouns? Are you asking others and sharing yours only in spaces with a queer audience? If so, work on that! (I definitely still am.) Same goes with bathrooms: Does your school allow everyone access to multistall all-gender restrooms? Start a petition, if not! Do your professors constantly divide classes into men and women for exercises or debates, erasing nonbinary students? Pipe up!

3. Advocating

Marginalized people are tired of advocating and speaking up for themselves, which is why it's so important for you and the rest of the community to rise to the challenge of supporting them. But first things first: You need to listen to others and educate yourself on your own. It is no one else's job to teach you. Seek out marginalized people telling their stories in their own words. "Maybe they're sharing stories about their experiences with law enforcement at school and the disproportionate amounts and kinds of discipline that Black students are experiencing. And that includes Black LGBTQ-plus students who can't separate race from sexuality or gender identity," Arredondo explains. So find out what activism exists at your school already (don't assume people aren't already doing this work!). Then find out what you can do to help those movements. Could your school look into restorative justice practices rather than highly punitive suspensions? Does your curriculum offer a broad range of work about and by people of color? Get information, and get involved. One of the biggest pitfalls allies can make, Arredondo adds, is assuming that you know what a marginalized group needs better than they do themselves.

When you do make your way into activist groups, queer alliance organizations, or other spaces in which you're not a member, don't take up too much space. Maybe this means you're a member of a committee working on a project and not the leader. Maybe it means waiting until all the marginalized people have shared first to ask a question. This is the work of decentering yourself so that you can truly be an ally who lifts others up.

This work has lasting effects. Take Marina, a resident adviser and recent graduate from a university in Pennsylvania. Early on in her freshman year Marina was coming to grips with her bisexuality. She was afraid to tell her family and didn't know how to broach it with her roommates, because even though they were accepting she was worried they would look at her differently. Eventually, she worked up the courage to talk to her own resident adviser, who was kind and supportive and pointed her in the direction of resources on campus, like the queer student union. "I think that she did a really good job of helping me come out to my friends and family, but also paving the way to make me a leader on campus in that community," Marina explains. In fact, her RA was so instrumental to her experience at school it made Marina herself want to be an RA, and she was able to help so many girls after her. Little things like offering support, affirming someone's identity, and being aware of your on-campus resources aren't so little to the people who need them most.

ℓℓℓℓ

If you're just starting to do this work: It's going to be okay. What we know about gender identity and sexual orientation may constantly keep changing, and it's all right to not necessarily understand or know everything. You don't *have* to know it all. Someone may describe to you their identity or attractions and it may make no sense at all in your head. That's okay. You don't have to be a scholar of gender studies to be there, to validate their identities and needs, and to do your best for your peers, especially if they're from marginalized groups. No one has ever kicked me out of their space for being incorrect about something (although who knows, maybe they wanted to!). If you mess up a pronoun, it's okay. Apologize without asking them to forgive you, and make a clear effort to work on it and do better. Because the most important thing is showing someone that you respect and affirm who they are. It's not about being perfect, it's about showing up for them.

7.

Staying Afloat in the Campus Fishbowl

How to Deal with the Pressures of Your New, Public, Private Life

If there was one thing I was wildly unprepared for before I left for college, it was the many ways in which dorming and campus living can make your private life all too public. Exhibit A: You may recall the "gentleman" I was briefly entangled with from chapter one. You know, the hockey player who told me I wasn't hot enough to have intimidated his penis into a state of flaccidity. One of the many red flags about that scenario was ignoring the age-old adage of "don't have sex with someone who lives on your dorm floor." Why? Because long after the sexy, fun times are through, you will have to bump into them doing every mundane activity you can possibly imagine for the next year. I thought I was prepared for the awkwardness, until one night after a big winter formal my freshman year. I brought a new guy home to my empty dorm room and we had sex—he did this move where he slid a pillow under my butt and it totally changed the angle and uunnhghgmmmm, was it good. Anyway, as I was walking him out, I realized that my first-week fling and a handful of his teammates were in the common room just outside my door. He made eye contact with me, shook his head, and chuckled. I hadn't done anything wrong, clearly, but he managed to make me feel like I had. I wasn't ashamed for anyone to know I'd be having more than just a couple sexual partners in college, but I wasn't prepared for people to directly assess those choices and deliver their verdict right to my face. As I huddled back in my room, I felt small and ashamed, too nervous to come out again and cross the hall for a glass of water.

DORMING DILEMMAS 101

College dorming creates this bubble in which you're dating, studying with, partying with, hanging out with, and casually screwing people who are in close proximity to you nearly all the time. Many universities have on-campus dorming requirements for underclassmen, so you'll be hard-pressed to avoid any awkward run-ins at all. But it's not just what people see that can make you feel like you're trapped in a bubble. It's what they can hear, too. In my case, it was a lot of unnecessarily loud sex for nearly a year. My sophomore year was a wild blur of making friends and making out with people at parties, but in my haste to enjoy everything around me, I wasn't paying attention to how it affected other people. Wrapped up in the glow of a new relationship, I wanted to show it off. I wanted everyone to know I was happy, desirable, and most important, having a lot of sex. Even though my new boyfriend and I both had single rooms in the same building, we wound up more often than not at his place. Little did I know how much our love life was torturing my boyfriend's suitemate, with whom he shared a wall. We'll call him Tom. Tom was the one who helped my boyfriend secure his own room when the dorm lottery rolled around—the latter had a bad "number," which meant he otherwise would have only been eligible for a double room. Using Tom's good number, they both got single dorms. As such, you'd think someone might be grateful for the help, or at least respectful of the person who liberated them from having a roommate as a sophomore. Early on in our sexcapades, Tom apparently let my boyfriend know he could hear us having sex pretty much all the time. In my case, this was largely due to a particularly theatrical habit of screaming at the top of my lungs—again, it was crucial that I let everyone know I was sexy and therefore having all the sex.

There was another more practical issue as well. My boyfriend's bed was aligned directly against the wall, which made any residual banging of the bedframe against the drywall reverberate even louder to his suitemate across the way. I had no idea at the time, but my boyfriend's lack of consideration for his suitemate put the nail in the coffin of their two-year-long friendship, and I was an active participant in the carnage. When we heard Tom thump his fist against the wall while we were going at it, my boyfriend and I just giggled. *Ha ha! Sorry about our crazy overactive teenage libidos!* It was a joke to me, a challenge, even. Being known as the girl having the craziest, loudest sex on the floor was a badge of honor. To this day, I'm not ashamed of that, but I *am* utterly embarrassed by how oblivious I was to Tom's side of things. I had a vague sense of some tension between Tom and my boyfriend, but that was all. So, at the risk of reliving some incredibly cringey moments, but wanting to better understand my impact on others during a somewhat selfish time, I called Tom. "I remember it being constant," he told me. To paint a picture: One time, when Tom's aunt called him to wish him a happy birthday, she commented on how the girl screaming in the background clearly must be faking it. Guilty as charged there, I'm sure. And there were times he wanted to hang out with his suitemate, but if he heard us in there, he knew there was little chance of seeing his friend until three or four in the afternoon. I blacked out a little from sheer mortification after Tom used the word "insatiable" to describe my sexual aura, but I soon came to and started to put it all together. Tom missed his buddy, and not only was their friendship changing, but it was changing in an unceremonious and rude way.

Tom had asked my boyfriend to move the bed off the wall. A simple request to mitigate the noise, but my boyfriend ignored it. Was it malice, selfishness, carelessness? I don't know for sure, but I know I never did my part to comply with his ask, either. While we were talking, Tom and I realized that, although we were friendly in college, too, we never spoke directly about the problem to each other. I wish we had, and while I didn't fully grasp the ways in which Tom was being insulted and ignored, I still knew enough to have been a better friend. I could have insisted we switch off whose room we went to each night. I could have helped rearrange the bed location in my boyfriend's room. I could have just dialed it down a few notches and left the *When Harry Met Sally* schtick out of it. But I didn't. Eventually, and for lots of different reasons, Tom lost patience trying to eke some compassion out of his friend. He filled out the paperwork to switch rooms and stuffed it in a drawer. They stopped talking and the friendship fell apart.

This story kind of sucks, right? If I'm being honest, I think the majority of the blame lies on my ex in this instance, but it's hard to look your past in the eye and know you could have been a better version of yourself. You will make a lot of mistakes in college, but walk into that dorm understanding that in a close community setting like the one you're entering, your private life affects more than just you and your partners. Don't be an asshole, and try not to have distractingly loud sex all the time. Prioritize your reputation for being a good person just as much as your reputation for being good in bed.

eeee

Lest you think I'm exaggerating the ways your intimate life can be put on display in college, just ask Marina, the former resident adviser we met in the last chapter. She was inspired to become an RA after seeing how expertly her first-year RA handled all the on-floor drama in her residence hall. Marina told me about a particularly upsetting dorm bubble incident. "My freshman year," she explained, "I ended up sleeping with a guy who lived directly across from me. Going into college, that is something everyone tells you not to do. And it just happened." Things might have been fine once they stopped hooking up, but this particular dorm had a culture of keeping room doors open, with roommates and friends walking in and out. For two straight weeks, her ex-hookup's squad would watch her walk down the halls when she passed by his room and would screech out his name at her in a stereotypically "girly" voice, or make moaning sex sounds. She couldn't escape. This was where she lived, and she needed to walk these halls every day. Make no mistake, this was harassment. It was terribly uncreative and boring harassment, but harassment nonetheless. Once Marina realized her ex was too much of a coward to intervene and ask his friends to behave like adults, she went to her RA, who promptly squashed it.

Marina watched these pressure cooker conflicts evolve as she herself became a resident adviser. She had to moderate a fight as one of her residents insisted on hours-long FaceTime calls with her boyfriend every night, keeping her roommate awake. (Yes, she refused to wear headphones.) And more shockingly, she dealt with a girl who heard her suitemate having sex through

There's no escaping it: Dorming opens your life up to prying ears and eyes.

the wall, recorded a Snapchat video with audio, and captioned it something to the effect of "when one of your roommates is having sex in the other room." Rightfully so, the girl caught in the background was livid, the one who took the recording claimed *she'd* been bullied, and ultimately rooms had to be reassigned. (I asked a lawyer about this, by the way, who explained that although video voyeurism laws vary from state to state, you might have a tougher time arguing a case with audio alone. Plus, if you're having incredibly loud sex, you may not have a reasonable expectation of privacy in the first place. While the student doing the recording was likely in violation of the school's code of conduct, it goes to show that dorming can put you in some truly unfair situations.)

Then there's Anna, who just graduated from a university in New York. She and her boyfriend were taking a break her sophomore year, and, as sometimes happens, Anna wound up getting briefly involved with a friend of her boyfriend's because, you guessed it: He was living on her floor. She was talking about it in a crowded dining hall when someone overheard, and told her on-again, off-again boyfriend at a party. Messiness ensued, and a lot of feelings were hurt unnecessarily. Anna knew she had to tell him, but she had hoped to find an ideal time when she could be open and honest; his being drunk in a frat house, told by a gossipy third party, was not what she had in mind. Campuses can feel incredibly small at times, even ones with thousands of students. Sometimes it will be a personal betrayal, sometimes you'll be the one in the wrong, but there's no escaping it: Dorming opens up your life to prying ears and eyes. So how do you manage? Here are some of the best tips from former RAs like Marina and other students who did their best to make it through.

Dorming Dos and Don'ts

1. Take your "roommate agreement" seriously.

It's likely that upon move-in, you'll be handed a document from the Residential Life office asking you and your roommate to agree on some basic points. How will you handle conflict? How will you keep the room tidy? What are your thoughts on visitors and overnight guests? RAs told me that all too often, roommates breeze through these as fast as possible, not taking the time to dive in and consider how they'll really feel in a moment of disagreement. Then later down the line, they're surprised when a fight breaks out and they're not quite as chill as they thought they'd be on day one. Really take the time to get into these discussions, even if you don't commit it all to paper for an administrator to see. Ask each other how many times per week you'd be comfortable being asked to leave so one of you can have the room for hooking up. Ask each other how much notice you'd need to vacate the space. What kind of social privacy do you expect from each other? If your roommate sees someone she knows leaving your bed in the morning, is that knowledge up for grabs to chat about at brunch, or do you want to hold each other to a certain standard of discretion? Get honest about how late is too late for audible laptops and phones, and be prepared to compromise. You may end up being awake a little longer than you wanted, or you may need to call it quits earlier than you think is fair. Invest in headphones and eye masks, but most important, be honest with your roommate *before* a problem happens.

2. Consider practical precautions.

Once you've gotten the go-ahead for a little intimate time in a shared space, don't forget obvious stopgaps: Lock your door! In speaking to current students, I heard several "I got walked in on!" horror stories that could have easily been avoided with a turn of the lock. I'd also advise adopting a "knock first" policy with your roommates. Yes, it's their space, too, and they're free to enter any time, but if they don't know whether or not you're alone in there, those few extra moments a knock affords can spare everyone an eyeful. Then there are more nuanced sex safeguards. Take for example, the humble shower-sex session. Super popular among college students, possibly because it's not something you could easily get away with when you were living at home (try explaining to Mom why you're saying goodbye to your boyfriend with wet hair right as she walks in the door), shower sex requires creativity. Audrey, a sophomore studying in Southern California, knows

> **If you want to speak for yourself, rather than having your sexcapades speak for you, plan ahead for privacy needs.**

firsthand. Audrey was hooking up with her best friend's suitemate, and when he suggested they get busy in their suite's showers across the hall, she enthusiastically agreed. In their haste, however, they forgot to plan ahead and realized that after they were done, there was only one towel hanging in the bathroom. Audrey wrapped herself up and trotted back to her hookup's room to grab another for him, as he waited shivering and naked in the shower, only to bump directly into her best friend . . . who had no idea she was having sex with one of his roommates. It was no big deal, just a little embarrassing, but drives the point home: If you want to speak for yourself, rather than having your sexcapades speak for you, plan ahead for privacy needs. And always bring extra towels to the bathrooms before shower sex.

3. Don't be afraid to ask for help.
The sad reality of joining any new cohort is that you may be forced to interact with those less kind, patient, empathetic, and mature than you. That last one is probably the most relevant in a college setting—your confidence might be betrayed, your privacy violated. It's not fair or right, but idiots cannot always be molded to act like fully functioning young adults. Guys will catcall and laugh, especially if they see your autonomy as a threat. Roommates, regardless of gender, will be cruel and cold. For better or worse, you all live in this community together. So if, like Marina, you feel harassed or even just overwhelmed with a situation, reach out to someone like an RA, dorm adviser, or trusted friend. If Marina hadn't done so when she was struggling with post-hookup dorm taunting, she may never have gone on to become an RA and help other students like her. RAs can help you navigate conflicts, even when it seems impossible. For those of you who are just not comfortable letting someone else in on the drama, my RA sources shared their best advice: Skip the passive-aggressive notes and talk face-to-face. Agree to put your phones away during the discussion so you can be truly

present and receptive to each other. Women especially, they noted, tend to be afraid to make their roommates mad or rock the boat, so we shrug off important conversations. Instead, be transparent about how you're feeling. As Marina put it, "I think a lot of conflict stems from the fact that you think that you know how the other person is feeling and you think that you completely understand their background, and you absolutely don't." Hear each other out.

⚠ **Don't let passive aggression and the fear of conflict prevent you from finding common ground.**

COLLEGE RELATIONSHIPS 101

Another Kind of Bubble

I am the last person on the planet to tell you not to get involved in a serious relationship in college. I've had spectacularly shitty relationships that messed with my self-esteem, and truly affirming, supportive partnerships that taught me how to care for another person. All of these experiences helped me learn more about who I am and what I wanted along the way. By all means, date away, but it's crucial to be aware of the ways in which a serious relationship can trap you in a bubble during your precious college years: a bubble of adoration, constant sex and feel-good hormones, but a bubble that separates you from the rest of your peers and potential experiences nonetheless. Think critically about if it's worth it.

All this got me thinking about my freshman-year boyfriend, Andy. There are few turns of phrase that can truly capture the all-consuming, inescapable, desperate feeling of being in love for the very first time. The world fades to a haze and a force field of rumpled bed sheets, soft kisses, and constant laughter envelops you and the only other person who seems to matter. You feel safe, understood, and held. But the protective embrace of a serious relationship isolated me. For a year, we snuggled in bed, ordering a truly unholy amount of Domino's, watched Netflix, and fell deeper into a trance. It was so intense that Andy would often get up in the morning, struggle to say goodbye before class, walk halfway there, and then return immediately, jumping right back into bed with me. (Let it be known that I was too much of a professor's pet to ever skip a class.) While many of my dormmates were off applying for research assistant positions and attending guest lectures, I was in a blissful daze that carried me from class to my new boyfriend's dorm, with no stops in between. Over the summer we house-sat his uncle's apartment in Brooklyn. We walked the promenade, stared at the city lights at night, and I got a taste of what it felt like to be an adult in love. When we returned to college as sophomores, however, we had both begun to wonder what it would be like to be single at school. A break turned into a breakup, and as I looked around at all the dynamic and fun social groups around me, I realized I hadn't taken the time to make any friends. I was alone, self-conscious about being alone, and had no idea where to start. I joined some clubs and eventually found the group of girls with whom I now celebrate promotions, weddings, and babies, but it took work. I don't regret a second of falling in love with Andy, but I often wonder what else I may have missed in my yearlong cocoon of takeout and TV.

Emmy, who recently graduated from the University of South Dakota, knows exactly what I went through. Emmy got serious with her boyfriend in her sophomore year of college, and once that happened, she estimates they were together 95 percent of the time. "We would take classes together if we could, we played video games together, we would cook together, watch movies—we were pretty much inseparable," she says. Emmy had friends who were getting married already, and she always wanted to walk down the aisle by the time she was twenty-five. So when she met her good-looking, wonderful boyfriend, she figured this was it. "Why would I want to go to parties and hook up with anyone when this relationship would be my long-term goal anyway?" she explained. But then something happened her senior year. Whereas previously she had spent her time with other partnered girlfriends, now Emmy started hanging out with some "female friends who were super independent, really sex positive, and didn't need a boyfriend." It threw her into a tailspin for her second semester of senior year. She suggested an open relationship to her boyfriend, but the situation quickly unraveled. She wanted more freedom and he was uncomfortable with it. "As I entered the adult world and left college, I didn't want to be tied down to one person, having to make plans around the two of us," she explains. It wouldn't be fair to boil Emmy down to a cautionary tale. Like me, she doesn't regret the relationship and feels it offered her invaluable support, but she admits she let it drag on longer than it should have, and knows she could have given her friendships a little more TLC than she did.

So how do you balance the desire to practice real intimacy with a beloved partner and not miss out on the once-in-a-lifetime social experiment of college? To start, I wish I had set better boundaries. Had I stopped to try even the most obvious of strategies to fix things, I could have applied a simple 1:1 rule to my socializing. For each weekend evening, I could have allotted one Friday for parties with classmates, and one for languishing in bed with my boyfriend. Even if we went out to parties together more frequently it would have helped broaden my horizons. Rather than shoving my own social life to the margins, I could have taken the effort to carve out moments in my week and keep them sacred and separate from relationship time. For example, a standing weekly lunch appointment with the cool girl in my Intro to Anthropology class. ⚠️ **Take the time to create those moments that are just for you, and keep to them as though they're an important doctor's appointment.**

Emmy also learned some concrete and useful lessons from her long-term college relationship. In addition to not letting anyone tell her that she "should" have reached a milestone like marriage by some arbitrary age, she set boundaries of her own. For example, when a position opened up at her on-campus job, her then-boyfriend expressed interest in it. But since they spent so much time together as it was, they decided it would be too much. This space, Emmy decided, should be kept as a place for her to nurture relationships with her coworkers and have some "her" time. Sound advice, indeed.

COLLEGE RELATIONSHIPS 201

Perspective and Balance

Sometimes it's challenging to figure out if your love–life balance needs work at all. To get some perspective, Greta Nielsen, MA, LCPC, NCC, a licensed psychotherapist and co-owner of Illuminate Therapy & Wellness in Palatine, Illinois, who works predominantly with adolescents, sheds light on the crucial art of balance. For one, she explains, it's totally normal for relationships at this time in your life to feel urgent. The adolescent brain has a tendency to focus on the present, and is excellent at identifying how you feel in the moment, but it's not always so great at forward-thinking, especially when it comes to the loss of ending relationships. "Nobody wants to be vulnerable enough to think of something that is that important to them, something that they feel so connected to, as a potential loss," Nielsen says. Young adults have a tendency to hang on in the here and now in order to beat back those fears, whereas older adults have an easier time sensing that the loss of a relationship isn't a loss of their whole identity.

To avoid losing yourself in a relationship, Nielsen recommends taking stock of all your different roles and identities, and who you spend time with to honor and fulfill those roles. A helpful metaphor she uses is to think about your life like spokes on a bicycle wheel. When all the spokes are present and properly aligned, you're in for a smooth ride. If not . . . you get the picture. Imagine your spokes as the different facets of your life: your physical wellness, your academic performance, your family relationships, your social life, etc. Then think about all of the people who help you flesh out those areas. If you find you're studying with your partner, going to the gym with them, only going to parties if they're by your side, or you don't want to go home for the holidays unless they're invited, too, your wheel is out of whack. No one is saying that's a sure-fire sign the relationship needs to end, but it's a sign that you're neglecting other areas of your life that will make it hard to cope without a little more balance. Look at those areas and ask yourself: Who else can help me even things out? Can I ask a friend to come to the library with me to prep for Biology exams? Can I sign up for a dance class and get my exercise while I meet new people? Slowly but surely you'll develop new support rods who can help you explore your identity as it relates to you, and not just to your partner.

The ramifications for not keeping your bike in check are real, Nielsen notes. For one, getting into a super-intense relationship early on in your college career, and being unable to find equilibrium, can stunt your social life, as I've mentioned. Freshman year is when a lot of social bonds are formed, she adds, and if you're coming late to the game it can dull your confidence to jump into the fray. That doesn't mean it's impossible by any stretch, just that it can be a bit trickier, and if you're feeling frightened off, you may be less likely to try. More long term, however, being unable to create healthy relationship boundaries can affect your life in lots of ways. Getting sucked into intense relationships that you don't have the control to balance can lead to anxiety and perhaps be connected to low self-esteem, Nielsen explains. "They're so focused on this relationship that they feel helpless and powerless to function without it. There's a lot of dependency which can be a self-fulfilling prophecy for their fears of abandonment." You become so worried someone will leave you because you cannot fathom other ways to meet your needs besides this relationship that you become overly dependent, which can tear apart even the best relationships—a terrible cycle that can ultimately lead to picking unhealthy and dangerous partners out of insecurity. If this sounds overly grim, take heart. Date long, date hard, but leave room in your week for time by yourself and time with others. If you can do that, you can do just about anything.

SURVIVING SOCIAL MEDIA 101

A Bubble about to Burst

Campus "bubbles" can make you feel trapped inside a system, unable to see out. But social media sometimes has a way of making us feel like we're trapped on the outside looking in. Although it wounds my aging pride to say it, when I was in college, all we had was Facebook. Even without the constant stream of updates and posts we're bombarded with today, I still remember the sting of finding out my friends went on a spring break trip without me when I saw the album they uploaded upon their return, full of gleaming sun and strappy swimsuits. Although we don't often feel that our peers are purposely leaving us out and broadcasting it on social, we feel the pressure nonetheless. Take Divya, a twenty-one-year-old senior at a large university in the Northeast. Especially when Divya was a freshman, she'd sit in her dorm room and look at everyone's stories on Instagram. Even though recent stories might be images and videos from ages ago that had been saved on someone's camera roll, or could have happened just a few hours earlier, when you're consuming them one after another in real time, it can give the impression that everything is happening all at once. For Divya, this made her feel as though everyone was out partying except her, and it was easy to lose perspective. "You don't individually break down that the person whose story you're seeing might have only gone out once that week," she says. But when you binge-watch a bunch of people's activities on your phone in quick succession, it creates this internal pressure. "Because you're seeing all these people out all the time, you feel like, *I have to be out 24-7*." Ultimately, Divya felt forced to be at parties all the time, even when she wasn't feeling well or had no interest in socializing.

⚠ **Don't get me wrong, a little encouragement to get out and about during the crucial bonding moments of freshman year isn't a bad thing, but if your body is telling you you're not up for it on any particular evening, it's probably for a good reason. You should *want* to explore your new social life, not let Mark Zuckerberg guilt you into it.**

Akane Kanai, PhD, a lecturer at the School of Media, Film and Journalism at Monash University, reminds us that we're not crazy if the internet winds up making us feel bad. She explains that even though social media sites can seem like a great equalizer, open to all and typically free to join, like-minded people have a way of finding one another and forming exclusive in-groups, whether through shared languages of internet humor or by posting status-signifying photos with their best friend. It's unsurprising that the downsides are real. Data suggests that those who are super plugged in to social media and feel emotionally invested in their feeds (e.g., using multiple apps for long amounts of time, constantly refreshing for likes, etc.), are at a higher risk for anxiety and depression. And if FOMO (fear of missing out) has you continually obsessed with your Snap streak, you're likely exacerbating those problems and feeding into the cycle.[1]

It's important to remember the early origins of social media, like Facebook, Kanai explains. After all, the early premise was assessing the attractiveness of Zuckerberg's female classmates and creating a network that relied upon the exclusivity of an elite Ivy League ".edu" address to join. Since then, it's no secret that social media prioritizes images of luxury and attractive bodies, which often translate to thin and white. It's essentially designed to facilitate ranking. Even if you're a member of these "desirable" groups—but especially if you're not—it can create a lot of pressure to live up to. Kanai adds that these apps are engineered to suck you in; their "constant connectivity" means that the never-ending updates of all your friends encourage you to use it daily, rather than just a few times a week. Those are some hard chains to break. So you're stressed, you can't put your phone away, you constantly feel like your life isn't as fun as the people's around you, you're inching toward social media burnout: What now?

For one, Kanai suggests, try and reframe your thinking. Social media is constantly pushing us to optimize ourselves, and so what you're seeing on Instagram isn't just your friends' and classmates' typical days. It's a handcrafted résumé, proclaiming: Here is me in my cutest outfit, in the best lighting, at my most flattering angle, having the most amazing time. It's not real life. Why should you compare your everyday self to someone else's perfected résumé?

If this thought exercise isn't enough to free you from your phone's beckoning grip, take an old study tip of mine: Use artificial means to lock yourself out from distractions. Willpower is overrated. Apps like SelfControl, Offtime, Flipd, and others can prevent you from opening certain time-sucking apps for a set period, giving you a chance to decompress, or even just finish a lagging homework assignment.

Finally, cut yourself some slack. Social media use isn't all doom and gloom. As some researchers note,[2] despite the moral panic many adults feel about our smartphones ushering in the downfall of humanity, social media can also be a strong community-building tool for marginalized groups like queer young adults who may face rejection at home. It can also be a key resource for seeking out information about safer sex practices, birth control, and more for people who don't have trusted sources growing up. All this to say, there is good and bad to just about everything in life, and the key is finding your own personal balance.

SURVIVING SOCIAL MEDIA 201

When the Digital Bubble Pops: Nudes, Sexts, and Revenge-Porn Safety

Digital mishaps will happen in college, especially since the dating pool is more concentrated than in postgrad life. Take Toni, a senior at a university in the South. She and her group of four close girlfriends will all periodically use Tinder at the same time. They swipe, match, and trade photos of the guys they're interested in. But it doesn't always finish with a Tinderella happy ending. "We'll talk about how cute he is and the things he says, and then we start realizing, *I think we're talking about the same person*," Toni explains. Then over group text, her friends will proclaim, "Everybody send a picture of him at the same time!" Only then do they realize they're sending different photos of the exact same guy, culled from different social accounts. To date, this has happened to the girls at least three times. Situations like these have a pretty easy resolution in Toni's squad, thankfully. If the match in question has been sending all of them the same exact messages, they'll all just cut off communication. If it seems like an honest faux pas of super enthusiastic, coincidental swiping, however, they'll decide who seemed to have the most chemistry, and the rest will back off.

But what about the less honest mistakes, the stories that don't make for laughs over brunch? A bit less than half of young adults eighteen to twenty-nine have engaged in some sort of sexting, be it explicit images or messages.[3] Unfortunately, however, 1 in 10 young women under thirty will experience threats of leaking those sensitive communications.[4] So how do you walk the line of participating in a practically ubiquitous foreplay tactic and keeping your private correspondence safe? First off, if you're under eighteen, or if you're over eighteen and sexting with someone under eighteen, the risks for sending nude photos are steep. If you're, say, nineteen and dating someone who is seventeen, possessing these images of a minor is considered child pornography, and is a federal offense. Thankfully, if you're both of age, you can use some common-sense strategies and digital security tips to keep your nudes just a little safer. Nicole Nguyen, a personal technology columnist, breaks it down. The downside, she explains, is that there's really no way to totally control the malicious intent of another person. You can't stop them from flashing their phone (and your pics) to their buddy, taking a screenshot or using another device to capture a disappearing Snap, or even save and repost your images out of spite if the relationship turns sour. So much of deciding whether or not you can safely sext someone comes down to trust, a difficult variable to quantify. My general guideline is that weeks is not an appropriate metric of time spent with someone before you can start sexting, and waiting until the month mark will help you get a better sense of character. Next, and while it may seem obvious, Nguyen recommends that if you're going to send nude photos, make sure you cannot see your face or any identifying tattoos, piercings, or markings. This little bit of plausible deniability can make all the difference in a worst-case scenario. If you never include those details, it's significantly harder to

100 percent prove it's you in a leaked photo situation. Next, she says, talk to your partner about what kind of privacy you expect with these photos.

Then of course there's the issue of keeping your photos safe from hackers, who have grown more and more sophisticated. Simple things like allowing photos you take on your camera roll to auto-upload to the Cloud could leave you vulnerable to hacking and phishing scams. Big companies like Facebook, which owns Instagram, pose a risk, too. "I think that essentially anything you upload to social media you should consider potentially public-facing in the event of a hack. Even things sent through direct message," Nguyen explains. "Because Instagram and Snapchat are accounts with usernames and passwords, they can be leaked onto the internet. People recycle passwords all the time, and there are data breaches happening very regularly. So if you reuse a password, then a data breach that affected your Coachella account from 2008 could potentially affect you today, because that means a hacker could open Instagram and guess your password." And . . . post your private information anywhere they wanted.

What about disappearing media like Snapchat and DMs? They're all potentially a liability, too. "That's private information that's proprietary to either Facebook or Snapchat. We don't know if that media is actually being deleted off of servers. And while I trust that they employ the brightest minds and their servers are safe, there's always the threat of a hacker or disgruntled employee getting into those servers, and that piece of media may exist somewhere deep in the ethernet of Facebook's back-end servers. Even though in your app it has disappeared, it's not entirely clear that it's completely evaporated from Facebook's systems." If I may, that's pretty fucking scary! My best advice? Steer clear of using social media apps to send nudes, because you just never know. Instead, she recommends using a messaging service with end-to-end encryption, meaning that even if hackers get in, they won't be able to decode your messages or photos. It's the difference between sending your note in a sealed envelope versus on the back of a postcard. Signal also offers tools that allow you to blur your face and has a camera in the app that won't save the photos you take to your camera roll. You can also adjust your settings to have the photos you send disappear after viewing, which may help reduce your chances of someone on the other end leaking it but again doesn't control for screenshots. Still, it's always wise to make sure you're not sending images that will live forever in someone's phone as a default.

Surviving Revenge Porn

Carrie Goldberg is a lawyer who owns a victims' rights law firm, C. A. Goldberg, PLLC. Goldberg deals with revenge porn cases—where someone nonconsensually shares nude images of another person—all the time. If you find yourself in that position, her advice is three-pronged.

1. Try not to panic.

This is an incredibly stressful situation, and it makes total sense that the first thing you might do is freak out. In the moment when it's happening, it's easy to feel isolated. But remember that you are not alone. "There are a lot of people who've been through it and gotten out the other side," Goldberg explains. You'll need as clear of a head as you can manage to navigate the logistics of what comes next.

2. Gather evidence and know your resources.

Goldberg says that while you might want to go on a deleting and reporting spree, take a beat and collect any evidence. Take screenshots of your material on whatever site you've found it, gather hyperlinks to both the material and your abuser's profile, and then follow any channels laid out for reporting violations on the site. If the person who did this to you decides to take it down right away but you still want to seek justice, you'll need evidence to prove it happened. Goldberg counsels that you can approach that end through the court systems and the Title IX office at your school, which deals with discrimination. She warns that while the criminal justice system moves slowly, you may have the option of getting an order of protection from a family court, which can in some cases be issued the same day. That, or a no-contact order issued by your school, can keep your abuser away from you, out of your classes, and out of your dorm.

3. Never try and deal with trauma alone.

These cases are fraught with emotion, and you need support systems to help you deal. Whether it's a friend, family member, school administrator, or therapist, make sure you've got people in your corner who will listen to you and be there for you.

ееее

In college, my friends and I used to get ready for parties and nights out at bars with a soundtrack of Ke$ha blaring in the background. We all loved the hits: "TiK ToK," "Animal," "Blah Blah Blah." But the earworm that stuck with me the most is her song that urges you to "Take it from a former overexposed blonde." While her lyric is likely an allegory about the all-consuming nature of the press when it comes to celebrity, it means something a little different to me when I think about it today. I've been that overexposed blonde. Not only in college when I invited the entire dorm floor into my sex life via cartoonish sex-screaming, but even after. When I first knew I wanted to write about love, sex, and relationships, I published some details I wish I had kept private. Things that will live on the internet forever, whether I like it not (and I don't). These are not life-ruining confessionals by any stretch, perhaps just . . . oversharing. Certain details in personal essays that I thought were fun and sexy at the time now seem gratuitous and unnecessary. This chapter, in a variety of ways, has been about privacy, both on- and offline. Your body and how you use it with others is nothing to be ashamed of. Just the opposite, in fact; it should be celebrated. But there's a fine line between celebrating and overexposing, and sometimes only time can teach you the difference. That line will be at different mile markers for each person and it will likely change as you reach different stages of your life, as it did for me. Hindsight has a way of altering your perspective on previous circumstances. As much as I'd like to say "take it from me," on this particular issue, I can't. So I'll say instead, think deeply and critically about what in your relationships is just for you, hold it close, and lock the door.

8.

In Your Head

How Your Mental Health and Your Sexual Health Are Connected

I was in a dressing room trying on clothes in Paris when I realized absolutely nothing in my usual sizes fit. It was on a summer vacation with my family just after my freshman year, celebrating my sister's college graduation, and I slowly realized just how much weight I had gained. At first I blamed petite European sizing, but after I caught glimpses of myself in mirrors and reflective shower doors, I finally stepped on a scale and saw that I was up about fifteen pounds (a number so comically on the nose for a freshman I didn't know whether to laugh or cry). I'd love to tell you that I simply didn't give a crap, and that

> **That's the thing about eating disorders: They're often unintentionally supported by those around us because our society is fatphobic.**

I went on my merry way without viewing my body as a problem to be fixed, but I did not. I couldn't tolerate it. I was physically and mentally incapable of accepting that people's weights go up and down, that bodies change with seasons, age, menstrual cycles, and so much more, and that there's no inherent moral value in being a smaller size. That moment in the changing room launched a summer of fairly extreme disordered eating, and left me with a decade-long struggle to accept myself without fixating on what I perceived as flaws, be they real or imagined.

When I got back to college for my fall semester sophomore year, people noticed I had lost weight—even more than I'd gained—and with all the extra attention it was hard not to believe that I had done something right. That's the thing about eating disorders: They're often unintentionally supported by the people around us because our society is fatphobic. And while I suppose I was winning superficial points with strangers, my relationships were feeling the strain. What unnerved me most about getting heavier was how it had happened slowly, seemingly under my nose, and yet I hadn't noticed until it hit me all at once. How could my body have been so far removed from my own control? I attempted to compensate by controlling everything (and everyone) else around me.

God forbid if my boyfriend suggested going out while I was chained to the elliptical in our dorm's basement. "Sorry, *I* want to take care of myself," I'd snarl in return, as though he were committing a doubly heinous sin by both attempting to stop me from working out and not exercising himself. With my family I was even worse. I'd have knock-down, all-out sob-fights if we planned to go out to dinner and I had deemed there was nothing on the menu I "could" eat. I wasn't doing it to purposefully punish my loved ones, though they may have felt otherwise. I just couldn't handle how helpless I felt when I wasn't able to control my body to my standards. So I lashed out often, trying to displace some of that inner torment onto others. Since then, my body image has been a near-constant third companion in every relationship I've had. More boyfriends than I can count have seen me break down, weeping about how a certain dress didn't fit right anymore or that I just hated the way I looked in everything. And nothing they could ever say or do could fix it, leaving us at an awkward standstill until I found something to throw on my body that didn't make me shudder when I looked in a mirror. I had people in my ear whispering conflicting messages all at once: *You look great. We're worried about you. You must be crazy.* Who should I believe? Some days I felt incredible, others repulsive, but mostly I felt alone. I didn't know then just how common these types of mental health issues were among women my age.

MENTAL HEALTH DISORDERS 101

They're So Damn Common

Mental health disorders in the college population are pervasive, with roughly 1 out of 3 freshmen suffering from at least one disorder.[1]

Another survey of 50,000 students of all years suggests 39 percent of students are "experiencing a significant mental health issue."[2] Complicating matters further, mood disorders like anxiety and depression are anywhere from two to three times more common in women.[3] Worse still, young adults in college often aren't getting the treatment they need. While the number of students with mental health disorders seeking treatment has increased over time, just 34 percent of those identified with disorders received treatment in the last year.[4] That means a lot of students are falling through the cracks. It's no small wonder Gen Z is most likely of all generations to report poor mental health.[5] With the constant threat of school shootings, the anxiety that social media can sow, climate change inching us closer and closer to destruction, not to mention global pandemics rearing their ugly head, I think it's fair to say adolescence has never been so daunting and complex.

It's also important to acknowledge the ways in which mental health issues can affect marginalized communities differently. Black youth today have come of age during a turbulent era when remote learning and school closures upended their education, as they simultaneously witnessed a string of police violence against people who look like them, a trauma unto itself. It goes without saying that the latter is not a new problem, and systemic racism can wreak havoc on mental health. LGBTQ teens report high rates of anxiety and fear, in large part due to threats of violence and lack of acceptance.[6] Also, global pandemic.

You're living through a lot, to say the very least. But staring at a laundry list of statistics doesn't always tell the full story. What impact does mental health have on your relationships? Your sex life? Your schoolwork?

EATING DISORDERS 101
Why They Thrive in College

When I first met Cara, a sophomore at a large university in California, she was striding into a study room in the library and telling off a guy in the firmest but kindest of terms. She had booked the space for us, and this guy was lingering beyond his time slot and playing dumb. Cara assertively and calmly told him what was what and that he needed to bequeath the room. He eventually scampered out. This stuck with me long after our chat, because the display of authority Cara presented felt just out of reach when we started talking about her history with eating disorders (EDs). She first became aware of the concept of calories, and how exercising could burn them, when she was in seventh grade. Since then, it's in her mind at nearly all the meals she's eaten. She then rattled off an estimate of roughly how many calories she'd eaten that day, and I felt an aching sadness wash over me. Because this beautiful, effervescent young woman made so much space in her mind for this restrictive behavior, yes, but also because I had also only eaten a small granola bar on the go after squeezing in a workout that morning, and it was far past lunchtime. I still wasn't taking care of *myself* the way I longed for Cara to tend to *herself*. We talk a bit about the freshman fifteen, and Cara interjects. "The freshman negative fifteen is also a big deal because no one's watching you eat. So if you have patterns of disordered eating, coming into college you can eat whatever you want. Or nothing."

I was taken aback by her bluntness and how sad it made me feel, but this holds up. Pamela Carlton, MD, who has decades of experience in pediatrics, adolescent medicine, and eating disorders, confirms that college is an especially risky time for eating disorders, for both those who have already been diagnosed and those who haven't. For the former, students may have been used to their parents ensuring they go to therapy by driving them to appointments, or modeling their necessary nutrition by making up their plates at dinner. At school, without those supports following through on their recovery and with the pressure of strangers watching them eat at mealtime, they may slip backward in their progress. This is why, Dr. Carlton adds, it's so important to have a plan in place with your care team before you go to college. For others who may be predisposed to eating disorders but have never had a diagnosed issue, the stress of school might propel them toward an ED. This, Dr. Carlton explains, is because eating disorders are maladaptive coping mechanisms—that is, a really unhealthy way of dealing with something upsetting. So when schoolwork, your social life, or anything else feels overwhelming and impossible to manage, some people reach for their eating disorder to reassert a semblance of control. Except the problem is, even if it may feel like it alleviates stress by applying order to your diet and exercise, it's incredibly dangerous. Anorexia nervosa has the second-highest mortality rate of all mental health disorders, second only to substance abuse disorders.[7] And some estimates suggest 32 percent of female college students have exhibited disordered eating or unhealthy weight loss patterns.[8]

EATING DISORDERS 201

How They Affect Your Relationships

Aside from physical complications, the mental and emotional impact of an eating disorder runs deep. As Dr. Carlton explains, it's easy for an eating disorder to impact your relationships. Bingeing-and-purging disorders like bulimia are likely to be associated with riskier sexual behavior, such as an increase in partners and a decrease in protection use. Restrictive EDs like anorexia can cause people to withdraw from their social lives and fixate on eating and exercise schedules. You might find it impossible to date if someone asks you out for a meal, for example, due to the stress of interrupting your own unyielding routines. You may also have a lower libido. Both types of disorders can cause an increased sense of secrecy (whether over an obsessive workout schedule or covert bingeing-and-purging habits), which doesn't lend itself to open and honest communication.

Then, of course, dating often means that someone will see you naked, a super-overwhelming and scary concept if you have an eating disorder. Cara knows that fear. She's not really into casual sex, and one of the reasons she cited was her ongoing struggle with body image. "It's difficult for me to trust someone enough for them to see me naked and touch my naked body," she explains. It takes her a while to warm up to physical intimacy, and even then it comes with its own challenges. With her current boyfriend, the first time they were about to get naked together represented a milestone, but not for the obvious reason. "The thing that I'm most self-conscious about is my stomach, my arms, my thighs, and my boobs," she told me. When her boyfriend went to take off her bra, it was nearly a nonstarter. He noticed her physical discomfort and they stopped to talk about it, and it was the first time she disclosed her body image concerns with him. While he was incredibly reassuring and they've since worked to build that extra trust and comfort someone with an eating disorder might need, there are days Cara doesn't want to take her T-shirt off around her boyfriend if she's even the slightest bit bloated. "That fear of rejection is always lingering. I'm worried that if I gain some weight or don't look super skinny one day he won't have sex with me. And I know that's not true," she explains. But that knowledge doesn't always quiet her anxious thoughts, and she hates when he touches her stomach.

⚠ Everyone is allowed to have preferences in the ways they want to be touched by their partners, but it might be time to get help if you have entire regions that are off-limits simply because you feel you're not good enough.

How Help Starts

Before you get treatment for an eating disorder, first you have to identify the problem. If you think you might be at risk, there are lots of online symptom-checker tools that can help, but you can also ask yourself some questions, Dr. Carlton explains. It'll be pretty obvious if you're bingeing and purging, but beyond that, are you avoiding situations that involve food? Do you overexercise? Do you feel so tied down by your exercise routine that it prevents you from doing something spontaneous? Mostly, she explains, you want to discern whether you control your food and exercise habits or they control you. (That second one is the "dangerous territory" category.)

What if you're worried about someone else? Unfortunately, data tells us that while colleges may offer services to those with eating disorders, they fall woefully short when it comes to screening for them.[9] There aren't a lot of opportunities for people at risk to be assessed and encouraged into treatment. This doesn't mean you should go running up to all of your friends who have fluctuating weight and scream at them about taking their illness seriously, but you may want to be aware of the signs. A roommate, for example, might be able to hear retching from the bathroom after meals. And they can also be on the lookout for what Dr. Carlton considers to be a key factor of eating disorders: rigidity. Does your friend's commitment to their routines make them unable to compromise on timing? Or overwhelmed, nervous, angry, or withdrawn when spontaneous plans are broached? It's important to know that it's not your job to "fix" someone else, and any adult with an eating disorder ultimately needs to be the one to get into treatment and commit to it themselves, but you can help by being part of their support system.

Giving and Getting ED Support

Whether you're a friend who wants to step up or someone with an eating disorder who wants to ask a partner or friend for help, here's what you can do.

1. Offer to go to a meal with them so that they can stay accountable to the nutritional plan their care providers have given them.

2. Help them fill the time they may have devoted to overexercising with other outlets, like studying or reading garbage magazines on the campus quad.

3. Communicate extra when it comes to sex. You may have to be more patient with someone who struggles with body image and you may need to let your partner know you feel vulnerable if you're the one struggling.

Ultimately, the biggest predictor of recovery for eating disorders is getting into treatment quickly, and not quitting early. If you think you're at risk, talk to your campus health office, a doctor back home, a parent, or anyone you trust who can help you get care. Building a team of friends and family around you, or being part of someone else's team, can help make the difference.

ANXIETY 101

It's Literally Everywhere

Why are mood disorders like anxiety so common in college? Jaycelle Pequet, LICSW, who works with lots of college students at their practice, the Institute for Emerging Adulthood, in the university hub of western Massachusetts, explains that at age eighteen and onward, you experience a big moment of transition. You may be leaving a familiar group, be it family, language, cultural community, and class, to move through this next stage of life that's often focused on your vocation—that is, what you want to do with your life to earn money as an adult. It's a lot of upheaval and pressure! And dorm life in particular can exacerbate it, Pequet adds. First, there's the constant stream of stimuli, whether on social media or the parties right outside your door. Then there's the expectation of growth and productivity in college, both socially and academically. The idea that you're there to make something tangible of your time in college, while rational on its face, can be daunting whether you're prone to anxiety or not. You may find yourself thinking: *What if I don't make something of myself? What if I do just okay in my classes? What if I only make a couple of friends? Will it be enough?* The notion of *OMG college, can't wait to have all my firsts and make this the best four years of my life!!* can be an unfairly high bar to set for yourself, even if you're excited for a seemingly good reason. Pequet adds that college isn't necessarily conducive to getting lots of rest and sleep, either, because of the aforementioned constant churn of schoolwork and socializing. It's a painful irony, because rest is one of many tools you can use to combat anxiety.

ANXIETY 201

How Anxiety Can Steamroll Relationships

Anxiety, Pequet explains, can increase your adrenaline and activate the parts of your brain responsible for breathing, heart rate, and so on—and it doesn't always leave space for rational communication. If you're in a relationship, anxiety might lead to increased fighting, withdrawing, and even a tendency to say or do things you might regret. For some, it may reduce libido, and for others it may kick it into overdrive. All of this unpredictability is not exactly a winning combination for smooth sailing in your relationships. Vivienne, a senior at an HBCU in the South has experienced anxiety firsthand—and so has her boyfriend. She first noticed it when she was a competitive cheerleader, before she got to college. The high stakes and pressure of a team sport, where one tiny mistake could cost the team a win, seemed to affect her more than her peers. She recalls being frozen before the routine started, shaking while she performed, and hyperventilating after it was over. "I was one of the top tumblers," Vivienne explains. "So if I fumbled the bag, that was it." Eventually, she realized it was more than just stage fright, as significant anxiety started rearing its head in other situations, like panic attacks in the middle of a test in class. For better or worse, her boyfriend understood what she was going through all too well. One night when Vivienne had a nightmare, a memory of a past traumatic experience, she found herself crying and hyperventilating in her dorm's bathroom. She called her boyfriend, and when she was so worked up that she could no longer respond on the line, he rushed over to her building. They hugged and, after he left, stayed on the phone until she could get her breathing under control and fall asleep. He knew what she needed and wouldn't let her feel alone with her discomfort.

While it might seem that dating someone who also lives with anxiety makes everything better, it's not that simple. Vivienne explains how she often finds herself comparing her situation with her boyfriend's, and worries her problems aren't as big or impactful as his. Her anxiety exacerbates these intrusive thoughts, and as you can imagine, this lends itself to some chilly conflict.

Marie Mizuno, LCSW, who works as a counselor on a college campus, agrees that anxiety, be it academic, social, or caused by a recent or past trauma, is a common concern among students she sees. It's not a stretch to see how trauma from the past can cause real problems in your romantic present. Take Marissa, twenty, who goes to school in Massachusetts. When Marissa was fifteen, she was sexually assaulted. Shortly after, she began to experience generalized anxiety and panic attacks a couple times a month. She also began self-harming. While the panic attacks were sometimes random, she often got them in the lead-up to a situation that might turn sexual. "I used to get pretty anxious if I thought that somebody wanted me in a sexual way. That would make me really nervous, because I'd think, 'Oh, well, I don't know their intentions. What are they going to do? What if I don't want them?'" Marissa says. With time, therapy, and the introduction of daily running and yoga, things have improved, but Marissa still gets a few panic attacks a semester. Most recently, she experienced one in the middle of having sex with her boyfriend a few months ago. She jokes that it was a "mood killer" but deep down understands how important it is to be with a partner who can empathize. She had wisely explained her history to her boyfriend before they started having sex, and so he knew what was going on when her body turned rigid and she had trouble breathing. He was clued in to her responses, stopped immediately, and talked her through it. In that moment, although they hadn't said

"I love you" yet, Marissa said she felt very loved.

It's convenient when a story wraps itself up with a nice little bow, but the reality is that working toward that kind of self-awareness and finding a partner who shares it is often a complicated journey. It sometimes feels like the world is conspiring against you. Like, oh, say, in a global pandemic that shuts down college and life as we know it for an extended period of time! Amanda, a junior at a medium-size university

> **If you don't have the tools to tackle mental health hurdles, it can be harder to keep yourself on track.**

in the South, dealt with the COVID-19 pandemic much as we all are: one frustrating, frightening day at a time. Amanda's brother has brain cancer, making him immunocompromised and especially at risk for COVID-19. And even though her school is doing some classes in person, thankfully her professors are letting her do as much as possible via Zoom to protect him. Still, her anxiety peaked. "I'm always worrying if it'll be normal again. And it really took a toll on my mental health. In the beginning when it was extra strict, I felt like I couldn't do anything; all my friends had to stay inside and stay home. And that one hit me a lot, because I'm a very social person. That was when my mental health was probably at its lowest," Amanda explains, in an all-too-familiar refrain. Complicating matters further, she and her boyfriend decided to move in so they could quarantine together, a step she admits she might not have made so quickly if it weren't for the pandemic. Like a lot of us, they found themselves navigating new conflicts. "We definitely get irritated with each other more because we're spending so much time together," Amanda confides. Still, it's not an insurmountable challenge. They take private TV and video game breaks to blow off steam, and they do the best they can. If you don't have the tools to tackle mental health hurdles, especially when the unexpected sweeps over the world, it can be harder to keep yourself on track.

How to Hold It Together When Everything's Falling Apart

Obviously, the answer is therapy. It's always therapy! But whether or not you go down that path, there are tools at your disposal that can help you navigate the choppy waters of your own mind. Here, Pequet and Mizuno share some of the strategies they use with their patients.

1. Know when to H.A.L.T.

Yes, that does mean "stop," and it's also an acronym for Hungry, Angry, Lonely, and Tired. When you notice you're overwhelmed and vulnerable, stop and check in with yourself. Are you feeling any of those four baseline feelings? If so, step back and make a decision to address it. If you're hungry, grab a snack. If you notice hunger is often at the root of some of your discomfort, try stashing granola bars in all your bags and coat pockets so you can get ahead of those hunger-induced spirals. Are you angry? If you can, try and pinpoint why, and even if you can't, stop and try a breathing exercise or a quick app-led meditation to calm yourself. Lonely? Call a friend, text your mom, draft an email, or better yet, stop and talk with someone IRL. Even a meaningless chat about the weather with a classmate can make you feel more connected if you've been feeling isolated. Tired? Take a nap if you can, or even just sit with your eyes closed for a few moments—and make a plan to go to bed earlier, too, duh.

2. Embrace the 20-minute break.

When you find yourself getting anxious and even verbally lashing out at your partner, separate from each other for twenty minutes. In that twenty minutes, the adrenaline and other chemicals that might be raging during a fight can come back down, allowing you to have a clearer head with which to deal with a conflict. Check in with each other. If you need more time than that—and you might!—take it. It's a lot easier to listen and communicate when you're not in a hyper-anxious state, and a break is a good way to get there.

3. Practice self-care you can do anywhere.

The "anywhere" part of this is key, because college often presents new and foreign surroundings. If your usual form of self-care is an extra-long bubble bath but your dorm doesn't have a tub, you might be feeling out of luck. Similarly, if the world has taught you that self-care means treating yourself to a massage but you're working part time to pay for your tuition, that's going to affect the way you spend money and put some forms of self-care out of reach. Try and practice self-care that's flexible and divorced from capitalism: free, and easy to do no matter where you are. Some examples: If you have a harsh inner voice, try thinking of someone who loves and cares for you. What would they tell you right now, if they could? Or if you find physical activity calms your thoughts, try finding private, picturesque spots on campus where you can take a walk. It doesn't matter how you practice your self-care, but it does matter that you find a way to keep it adaptable so you have resources to draw on in unpredictable circumstances.

4. Be direct with partners.

When it comes to talking about your mental health and how any particular condition or illness impacts you, do your best to be clear by using "I" statements to convey your feelings. Also, let them know exactly

what you need from them! Even if you don't have specifics, your partner should approach you with a willingness to listen, empathy for what
you're dealing with, and no defensive attitudes when you're sharing
how you feel. And if they don't know, tell 'em so.

5. Reframe negative thoughts.

Even if you're having garden-variety stress or anxiety about something
as straightforward as how you're doing in school, you can relieve a lot
of that internal pressure by rethinking your response to that worry. For
example, if you didn't do as well as you wanted on a test, instead of
convincing yourself that you're a failure, try reminding yourself that,
hey, you studied a lot and it was just a difficult exam. It happens. You
lived, and you'll live even if it happens again. Getting yourself to a place
where you can acknowledge that you're doing your best, and valuing
that just as much as if not more than a letter-grade outcome, can give
you a framework to think about stressors in a more productive way.

Okay, but What about Sex and Anxiety?

We've talked a lot about how mental health disorders of all kinds can
impact relationships, and sex, too, but hey, this is mostly a book about
sex. And you need sex coping strategies. From years of writing about
sex, research for this book, and—let's be honest—personal experience,
here's how to feel a little bit more like yourself when your head is messing with your body.

1. Don't have sex.

If you're not feeling it because of anxiety or depression, the worst thing
you can do for yourself (and the person you're doing) is to force yourself to be intimate. You're unlikely to have a good experience, it'll breed
negative associations with sex, and any halfway decent partner would

probably feel mortified you were having sex with them out of obligation. Trust your body when it tells you, "Hey, no."

2. Find ways to feel sexy by yourself.

Again, because mental health conditions and the meds associated with alleviating their symptoms can flatten libido, it's important to find ways to feel connected to your body. That may start with a simple yoga class or daily stretching, but to get in touch with your sensual side (it's still there!), try investing in an exciting new sex toy, or digging out some of your favorite lingerie that you usually save for special occasions. It's like in the airplane safety videos: You have to turn yourself on first before you turn on others.

3. Safe words, seriously!

Since anxiety and past trauma can impact your ability to communicate clearly, especially when you're agitated, try safe words. Yes, even if you're not into kink or BDSM, having a mutually agreed-upon word that means "stop, too much" can help send a message to your partner, even if you can't totally articulate why you're feeling that way in the moment.

4. Don't let yourself feel left out.

In college especially, it can often feel like the social activity of every weekend is to get laid. We swipe on apps to meet people, we beg our friends to introduce us to their hot lab partner, we go to bars, parties, and mixers to see if the next stranger through the door might be the one. Even when we all strike out, sometimes the most fun part of the night is reuniting back in a friend's dorm to rehash the ones that got away. But if mental health has suddenly put a damper on your desire to be intimate, especially if you were used to enjoying an active libido in the past, it's easy to feel left out. So remind yourself: There's no moral victory in having sex. And it doesn't mean you can't still enjoy parties!

Dance, chat, eat snacks, drink, or don't. Give yourself little missions for each night out that don't revolve around hooking up, like: I'm going to get to know that cool girl from French class better. I'm going to be a wingman for one of my friends tonight. I'm going to finally master a cut crease on my eyes. Whatever it is, reminding yourself that there are so many ways to have a full and active social life that don't revolve around sex will convince you that you're honestly, truly, not missing out.

5. Capitalize on the moments when you *do* feel turned on.

I used to think that sex was meant for certain times of the day: morning, when you wake up naked next to someone you've just started seeing and you can forgive the bad breath; or evening, after a night of party-ing—either bringing home someone new or rushing back to the person you wish you'd spent the night with in the first place. Then I realized I was missing out on oh-so-much sex if my "normal" windows of oppor-tunity were thwarted by feeling tired, out of place in my body, or just not into it. Especially in long-term relationships, sex can easily dwindle. It doesn't mean it will, but busy schedules, mounting responsibilities, pressure at work or school, lack of novelty can all wreak havoc on your sex drive. So if you're feeling horny at 1 PM on a Sunday, even if it feels out of nowhere, go to town. Don't let a missed opportunity of arousal go to waste waiting for a perfect time. Carpe do-'em.

What If Therapy Isn't an Option?

We all know what to do in a perfect world, but college is, for better or worse, imperfect. One common roadblock noted by students and pro-fessionals alike is the barrier to therapy on campuses. This is not to knock the excellent care providers and all the services they do offer, but in reality they sometimes fall short. Several of the women I spoke with admitted they stopped going to therapy for a variety of reasons, even when they knew they would be better off staying in treatment.

Some schools offer programs that cap at just a handful of free sessions. Some students don't feel comfortable getting therapy because they're on their parents' insurance. Some face wait times that render campus services unusable. Some can't afford to see a local provider in town because they don't have the money, or don't have access to transportation. And some just get overwhelmed navigating the complicated system of health care and stop trying. It doesn't matter why, but it's important to acknowledge the reality that ongoing therapy isn't always possible in a college setting. So what can you do if you've blown through your campus offerings and are in between options? Don't give up, and try these tips to get you through a transition.

When it comes to protecting your health and getting the care you deserve, you have to be your own advocate.

1. Ask your immediate resources for other options.

Don't be afraid to press your existing primary care physician, current therapist, or the campus mental health office for more information. They may have connections with providers elsewhere who can offer reduced rates on a sliding scale. You don't know what doors are open to you until you start wiggling all the knobs. The phrase "I am in crisis and need help I can afford" might become your best friend.

2. Have a point person for support in the interim.

Tell a friend or family member that you're having trouble accessing the care you need, just so you're not shouldering the additional frustration alone. This doesn't mean they become your de facto therapist, they're just someone who will now be primed to know you may need to talk some things out from time to time or that you might benefit from a check-in.

3. Consider a text-based therapy service to hold you over.

Some people believe in-person therapy is best, but lots have found success with app-based care, which can be done via video or text. A lot of providers have extended their services to include remote options due to the pandemic and many may continue to offer this type of expanded access after the fact. Sure, it may not be your perfect cup of tea, but it could offer some much-needed temporary support in the interim, most likely at a lower price point.

The most important thing is not to give up. When it comes to protecting your health and getting the care you deserve, you have to be your own advocate because no one will fight for you harder than you can. Don't quit; your mental health is worth it.

ﻉﻉﻉﻉ

Struggling with your mental health is common, but just because something is common doesn't mean you can laugh it off as inconsequential. Because I was medically stable, no one ever pushed me to get the help I really needed with my disordered eating. I desperately wish they had. In my early twenties I tried working on it with a psychotherapist. To start, we went through what I was eating in a day. When she told me that two eggs was "a lot" for breakfast, I knew I wouldn't make much progress with her, and I stopped trying. I let my life be dictated by numbers on a scale for so many years, it's at once humiliating and tragic. I look at pictures of myself from ten years ago and think, *How could this girl have hated the way she looks here?* Since then, I've seen other therapists and found medications that help with my anxiety. It's not perfect. Like the young women in this chapter, I've fallen in and out of therapy. But along the way, I've learned how to turn away some of the intrusive negative thoughts about my body.

Like millions of Americans stuck at home during quarantine and deprived of the gym (my personal church), I gained some weight. I'll be honest, I don't feel totally neutral about it. There is no point in sugarcoating my way into a happy ending for me and my body just to neatly close out this chapter. But it's okay, because I'm not letting it work me into a tailspin of doubting my self-worth. Instead, tired of feeling uncomfortable working from home in clothes that felt just a smidge too constricting, I bought two new pairs of jeans from a brand I love—one size up. They arrived in the mail, and when I put them on, I didn't feel like a failure. I just felt like me, except in pants that fit.

9.

Parents and the Politics of Sex

Practical Advice for Developing Autonomy

It may or may not surprise you to know that I never received an actual "sex talk" from my own parents. Not even little teaching moments along the way. Perhaps (but hopefully not) like you, I just got a series of not-so-subtle messages that I wasn't supposed to be having sex at all.

The first time I can recall getting the "sex is bad" message was when I was fourteen. I had started getting my period a year or two earlier, and the pain from my cramps was out of control. I did my best to get ahead of it, taking an Advil or Tylenol the very second I thought cramps might be creeping on, but if I was even a few minutes too late they'd balloon out of control. Doubled over a toilet in agony, I'd face intense, nausea-inducing pangs for hours. Though it would only take me out of commission for a day or two each month, no one wants their teenage daughter to be in pain, let alone pulled out of school because of painful periods. So my mom took me to the doctor, likely my pediatrician at the time, to talk about my options. When he suggested birth control pills, which would give me lighter periods, lessen the severity of my cramps, and make my cycle more predictable, I was on board but my mother was instantly skeptical. She asked if there was anything else, and my doctor shrugged and spelled out that unless she wanted her teenage daughter on habit-forming prescription pain meds, this was the best option. Miffed, she turned to me and said, "I just want you to know going on the pill isn't an excuse to start having sex."

The main reason you can remember something that happened at fourteen when you are currently easing into your thirties is that it had an impact on you. That one sentence contained so much subtext: that I shouldn't be having sex, so it must be bad. That if I *did* want to have sex, I couldn't do it just because I wanted to—I needed an excuse to rationalize it. That my need for a certain medicine was a problem that came with a warning, because it was associated with sex.

The situation did not magically improve a few years later when I did start having sex. I will not force you to sit through the details of my first awkward attempts at intercourse yet again, but to this day I'm still proud that I felt more or less prepared for it. I waited until I was seventeen—even though I had opportunities earlier, it never felt quite right, and I took that hesitancy seriously. I had been getting to know and trust my then-boyfriend for almost a year beforehand, and we used two forms of protection. A parent, I figured, could do a lot worse than me in terms of their child's sex responsibility–taking habits!

But the icy cold war between me and Mom didn't start the first time I actually had sex. It was months later, when she finally figured it out. I had been staying with my then-boyfriend at his grandmother's house in western Massachusetts over the summer. We were having lots of fun (and, in all honesty, lots of sex), so I called to see if I could change my bus back home to a later date. My mom freaked out, saying something to the effect that this

> **When you enter college, there is no shortage of conflict when it comes to independence, sex, and your family.**

wasn't just an endless sex vacation with no return ticket. I don't know why it set her over the edge, but after I got home she wouldn't talk to me for a few days. Then we resumed our normal mother-daughter relationship like nothing had happened.

It shouldn't shock you that our ability to communicate about sex didn't improve in college, either. Once, after a string of UTIs and yeast infections, I went to health services at school to figure out what was going on, and if it was somehow sex related. I called my mom and let her know what was up, to which she replied, "I wish you would be more discerning about your partners." I was crushed. I had come to her with a problem, and somehow she had managed to make it my fault. And sure, new partners and frequent sex can be risk factors for UTIs,[1] but this wasn't a "fault" situation. Was I sleeping with assholes and jerks who did not particularly care for my emotional well-being? Yes! Did they trigger UTIs and yeast infections on purpose? No! In just three exchanges, from adolescence to college, I got the message: I couldn't talk to my mom about sex. Not really, not if I didn't want to be judged.

When you enter college, there is no shortage of conflict when it comes to independence, sex, and your family. Why? And what can you do about it? Read on.

SEX TALKS 101

Why It's So Damn Hard for Parents

The obvious reason parents avoid "the sex talk" is because families don't much love thinking about one another as sexual beings, especially children. After all, do you relish sitting down and having a nice, long think about your parents getting it on? (You do not.) But it goes so much deeper than that. If you've ever felt annoyed or let down by your parents' hesitancy to be forthcoming about sex, you're not powerless to address it. The first step toward navigating just about any conflict is understanding where they are coming from. Melissa Pintor Carnagey, LBSW, founder of Sex Positive Families, an organization that helps families raise sex-positive kids, breaks down some of the reasons.

1. Their parents didn't have the talk with them.

Whether because of generational gaps, cultural upbringing, or some other reason, it's plausible that *your* parents never spoke openly with *their* parents about sex. If they didn't have those kinds of talks themselves, they don't necessarily have a model about how to start them with you.

2. Their school didn't have sex ed.

It's also likely your parents didn't have inclusive, comprehensive sex ed at their school either. So if they didn't hear about it at home, there's no guarantee they had the opportunity to learn elsewhere. Again, it's harder to duplicate a tricky situation you didn't experience.

3. They may have experienced trauma or sexual assault in their past.

"Parenting can be super triggering. Even if you thought you'd gone to therapy for that, you become a parent and your child enters certain milestones that can trigger some abuse or trauma that you experienced around the same age," Carnagey explains. Talking about sex could be particularly painful in that regard, and they may want to shy away from it altogether.

4. The stigma around sex is still so prevalent.

Sex is not one of those universally accepted topics we can chat about like the weather ("Nice orgasm we're having today!"). And because of that, we tend to be more secretive about it, like avoiding conversations or using euphemisms to talk about our bodies—think: saying "lady parts" instead of "vulva." Because it's considered taboo, sometimes parents just don't want their daughters having sex, period. They rationalize that if they withhold information about it, you just won't do it in the first place. Wrong!

I don't mean to absolve parents of their responsibilities to you, but it's important to try and cut them some slack while you push for the information you need—we don't always know what our parents are going through. To be clear, none of these reasons is an excuse for leaving a child in the dark about sex, especially since we're hungry for the information. A report from Harvard University showed that 70 percent of adolescent respondents wanted more information about the emotional nuances of romantic relationships from their parents.[2] This desire is complicated by the fact that half of all teenagers feel uncomfortable talking about sex with their parents.[3] Since not all parents are up to the task, and not all young adults are willing to get their sex ed from their parental units, we've got you covered.

SEX TALK 201

What's at Stake When We Fuck It Up?

Indulge me for a moment while I share some things that may or may not feel like a big old "duh" to you. Growing up in a sex-negative household, where sex is considered to be wrong or unacceptable or dirty, or even in a house where sex is completely ignored and avoided, can have lasting impacts, especially on young women. Dr. Lisa Damour, psychologist and bestselling parenting author, explains the general differences in the ways we approach sex with girls and boys. It boils down to what she calls an "offense, defense" discussion. For boys, we put them on the offense. According to Damour's summary of research on the topic, we tell boys, if you're going to have sex, wear a condom. That's it! On top of that, more than half of adolescents in one recent survey claim their parents never spoke to them about basics like how important it is not to pressure someone into having sex with you, how you shouldn't keep asking someone to have sex if they've said no, and how you shouldn't try to have sex with someone who's intoxicated.[4] Call me crazy, but I feel like these two things are related!

Girls, on the other hand, are put on the defense. We feed them a lot of "don't"s. We tell them don't get an STI, don't get pregnant; basically, don't have sex at all. And if any of those things *do* happen to you, they'll be your fault, because you're the one who went and had sex after we told you not to! This creates a culture of shame surrounding sex that women feel more profoundly than men. Damour adds, if you feel like you're not supposed to be having sex, you may feel more shame if you do have it. If you're feeling shame, you may be less likely to take care of yourself when it comes to getting birth control, STI testing, and more. This shame also contributes to young women sometimes feeling that getting drunk to have sex provides reputational cover, according to Damour, allowing them to disavow it later and brush it off as, "Oh it wasn't me, it was the booze." Unsurprisingly, this mentality can negatively impact your health over time.

Kacey, a sophomore who goes to school in Kansas, was raised in a conservative Christian family whose faith intensified when her father became actively involved in a strict new church. Although she says she was always close with her parents, it was a different story when it came to sex. "We didn't talk about it. It was just assumed that you don't do it. I never got a sex talk," Kacey tells me. The only time her parents did bring it up was when they'd gossip about another girl from town who got caught sneaking her boyfriend into her bedroom. You can imagine those conversations were not all that kind to the girl in question.

It only got worse when Kacey went away to college. During her freshman year, Kacey was sexually assaulted. She struggled with what that meant with regard to her faith, and wanted guidance. "How do you redraw your boundaries after a line has been crossed?" she wondered. But she knew she couldn't ask her parents, explaining, "They'd probably consider that a sin."

The trauma of enduring an assault is steep enough on its own. Imagine how unscalable the cliff would seem if you knew you couldn't get help from the people who are supposed to love you the most, because their first reaction would be to blame instead of soothe. I don't know Kacey's parents; I can't say whether or not she's right about them. But they've given her every reason to believe she's right.

To any stray parents reading this chapter, trying to suss out whether this book is right for your daughter: If you want her to come to you in her darkest hour, help her believe that she can. Tell her so until she knows it in her bones. She needs to know that you would never put your beliefs or your anger over loving and supporting her.

When Kacey did feel ready to have consensual sex with her boyfriend of a few months, she didn't know where to start. She realized everything she knew about sex either came from shoddy public school sex ed or from her assault. Even taking off her shirt was a struggle. "It was a very long process for me simply because I felt so ashamed every single time we would try and do anything," she says. Ultimately, she found her bearings by reminding herself that it's okay to feel awkward, that sex isn't like what you see in the movies, and you can take as long as you want until you feel comfortable.

Nora, a junior at an HBCU on the East Coast also knows what it's like to not be able to let her family in on her life. She was raised Christian and taught to believe that she shouldn't have premarital sex. As she reached high school, Nora started to realize that she's attracted to both men and women, and had trouble squaring her identity with what her church told her was and wasn't okay when it comes to relationships. One day, she decided to dip her toe into the waters of telling her parents and decided to "prank" them by telling them she was bisexual, just to see how they'd react. It didn't go over well. Her mom even started crying. From that moment on, she knew that this part of her identity is something she wouldn't be able to share with them. If that was a test, "They got a zero percent. *Let's retake the class and talk next semester,*" Nora quips. She knew she'd only try again if she were dating a woman and things got really serious, like if marriage were in the picture.

The Role of Mentors and Other Support Systems

The hard truth is that some parents can't be everything for you. We'll talk more about communication strategies a little later, but for some, it may just be that one of the best courses to take is accepting that your parents can't be everything for you. That doesn't mean you completely give up on their supporting you in other areas, but accepting that they won't change can free you up to seek out other people to support you and fill in the gaps your parents left behind. Kacey, for example, knew that part of being sexually active meant taking care of her sexual health, but her parents had expressly forbidden her from going on birth control. Without other options, she had to get creative and she started opening up to other people. Kacey works an off-campus job as a waitress on top of her schoolwork, so one day she asked an older coworker, who she calls her "second mom," how to get birth control. The coworker pointed her to student health services, where Kacey pays fifty dollars for her pills each time she needs a refill because she's afraid to run it through her parents' insurance. She knew they might find out what she's using it for. It hurts that she has to jump through these hoops because she can't rely on her parents, but she's grateful for the friends and coworkers who've become de facto mentors. (And just a note: There may be other free clinics nearby that offer reduced rates on birth control. If your campus health office quotes you too high a price, ask them where else you might be able to go.)

Nora, too, knows her parents struggle to accept anything outside of the heterosexual norms in which she was raised, but she doesn't see her situation as particularly tragic.

Your parents can't be everything for you.

She feels lucky in a lot of other ways that matter. In college she was able to explore intimate relationships with women more deeply and make friends who are bisexual. Meanwhile she appreciates how supportive her parents are of her academic goals. Plus, she has three siblings who love and accept her, and she focuses on the network of support they've built for one another over the years by shouldering the confessions and celebrating triumphs they don't think their parents can handle.

Sabra Katz-Wise suggests that—especially when it comes to queer students—don't assume all the doors to your family are closed forever. If you have a horribly rejecting family who kicked you out of the house and can't see you for you, yes, it's possible they will never come around. That'll make it extra important that you fill your circles with others who love you. But Katz-Wise notes that many families do in fact change their tune. A sibling who stands staunchly on your side might help a parent open their mind. Or, as Katz-Wise explains, that understanding may come as you reach certain milestones in your life. They might soften when they see how truly happy your partner makes you. "Some people in my circle came around when my wife and I had a child, and they started to understand a little bit more," she says.

Finding a Mentor

How do you get a mentor of your own to answer your tough questions or just let you be you? The best part is you may already know them. The same way you might get a promotion for excellent work at the office, you can decide to promote people in your life into bigger support roles. When you go away to college, you may find yourself leaning more on a sister, cousin, or aunt for advice. If you're unsure how to approach them, try kicking off those conversations with, "I have something on my mind and I really need to talk it out with someone. I know we haven't

> **In college, you get to rewrite any messages you've gotten about sex that don't feel right to you.**

always talked about these kinds of things, but I've always considered you to be open-minded, smart, and understanding. Would that be okay?"

Or you may find that the therapist at your school's counseling office really lifts you up and makes you feel confident in ways you never have before. You may make a friend who will hold your hand and drive you to the doctor to get an IUD inserted, or have an abortion, when you know your parents may not have done the same. Plus, as Melissa Pintor Carnagey notes, you may have mentors and support systems that you never even meet. Well-vetted websites like Scarleteen can fill in knowledge gaps and make you feel seen and certain social media activists can do the same by shedding light on topics you once thought were shameful. (When it comes to medical advice, however, you should only be listening to your doctors.)

College is a wonderful time and space where you get to rewrite any messages you've gotten about sex that don't feel right to you. Go ahead and build up your team of editors to help!

When Parents Get the Sex Talk Right

Okay, so we've been through some scenarios that I can safely categorize as "kind of a downer." But what might our attitude toward sex look like when we get to college if our parents did their best to be open-minded and informative? Lily is a sophomore who goes to school in Florida, and even though her parents aren't perfect, she's always felt okay—if not totally comfortable—telling them what's on her mind. From a young age, she remembers her parents being pretty open with her about sex. She didn't get one big sit-down sex talk, but lots of little lessons along the way. One time, when she was about nine years old, Lily remembers watching the movie *Grease* with her mom. She was really confused about the scene at the drive-in movie, where Danny puts his arm around Sandy, grabs her boob, and Sandy gets upset. So Lily's mom explained that some people like to touch breasts because they think it feels good, but that no one should touch hers unless she wants them to and tells them it's okay, and that's why Sandy was mad. Lily's mom didn't shame the act of boob-touching when done appropriately, plus gave a healthy lesson on boundaries and consent. Pretty easy!

Years later, when Lily wanted to buy a vibrator and was looking for some guidance, she went to her mom. They sat down and talked about it. Her mom shared that she masturbates, and probably did it even more when she was around Lily's age. Then she said that she was glad her daughter would have this as another option to make herself feel good, because she thought it was a healthy alternative to going out and having sex with someone just for the sake of an orgasm. After all, a vibrator on its own can't get you pregnant or give you an STI. She didn't want her daughter to depend on anyone else for sexual pleasure. Then, of course, she gave Lily the typical mom advice of, "Don't forget to clean it." Perhaps what I love most about this exchange is that Lily remembers it as a little awkward. Good! These conversations might always be a little uncomfortable because they revolve around topics we don't always feel like we can discuss freely. That's okay! It's important to have realistic expectations of how these talks will go. The discomfort is temporary; the effects can last a lifetime. Lily sees that now in her peers, and doesn't really know what to make of it when some of her friends have confessed that they think masturbation is unnatural and you should never talk about it. (Hint: Her friends are wrong!) She's grateful that she doesn't have the same hang-ups around intimacy as they do.

Lily isn't having sex yet, a combination of being a self-described late bloomer, having a slow discovery of her sexual identity, and the pandemic messing up her school year, but she feels comfortable with the idea of having sex eventually and knows exactly what qualities matter to her in a partner. Her family's acceptance has a lot to do with that.

AUTONOMY 101

Why It Matters

The transition from high school to college is a big one for both you and your parents. It's a moment where you have to start taking care of your needs and practice autonomy. It's the start of something exciting for you, but it could feel like the end of something to them. Are you the eldest child? They've never done this before! The youngest? You're their last baby going off to school! As always, a gentle reminder to cut your parents some slack during this transition. But like all changes, it goes smoothest when both parties are on board with how your relationship might differ going forward. So what does it mean for parents to treat their young adult children like, well, adults? It can look a few different ways.

Kim Cook, RN, a health and sex educator, thinks parents' instilling that sense of adulthood has a lot to do with how they engage with you on a day-to-day basis. For one, parents have to let kids develop their own ideas freely, without overly critiquing them. If you're home on a

If you want your parents to see you as an adult, you need to show them you're up to the task of acting like one.

break trying to tell your parents something you learned in a lecture at school, they shouldn't immediately start correcting you, even if they're not sure that you've got all your facts straight or if they disagree. (Obviously, this would not apply if someone was parroting back bigoted, harmful, or incorrect rhetoric.) Rather, parents might ask follow-up questions to go a little deeper on what you're thinking and how you formed your opinions. Even if they're getting more hands-off, parents can still show adult children they care by proving that they listen when you talk about your social life. Asking how your friend Rebecca is doing or inviting your new partner over for dinner goes a long way to showing that they respect the individual life you've created outside of the family. I had a lot of boyfriends in college and beyond, and bless my parents, they welcomed each and every one even if they knew it wouldn't last. I appreciated it in the moment and even more looking back, because it made me feel like an adult.

A Note for Parents

For any parents reading this book before giving it to their kid, if this advice is freaking you out, here are some tips to help you give your kid more autonomy. According to Dr. Damour, a perspective shift might help. Try to look at yourself as more of a consultant than a boss: Your children are not your employees any longer, but they might need to bring you in for help every now and then.

- Let your kid be in charge of their own health by booking doctor and dentist appointments. You might have done it for them in the past, but now you can remind them and show them how to do it on their own, rather than just doing it for them.

- Let your kid develop their own notions. After all, other adults don't routinely go around dinner parties patronizingly interrupting each other if they have a competing thought. They smile and nod and agree to disagree. And hey, maybe what you were taught when you were younger isn't necessarily true anymore.

- Stay out of your child's sex life. As with your own, it should be private, and is absolutely none of your business.

- Carnagey, perhaps, says it best: "If you want to stay connected with your children, create and maintain space that feels inviting and open and not judgmental. A space that's not about control or rooted in trying to control their outcomes."

Autonomy in Practice

It's important for you to know what autonomy can look like in practice—especially if you don't feel like your parents are letting you grow. That way, you will have specific points you can bring up with them on what you'd like to improve, rather than a blanket, "Ugh, you don't respect me!" which rarely goes over well. But it comes at a cost to you, too. Bree, nineteen, told me about the time in high school when her parents wanted to join a family-protection app that lets parents track their kids' phones, with super-specific details like how fast they're driving. She told them it felt like an invasion of privacy that made her uncomfortable. There was no reason for them to know where she was at every single second of the day, she argued. So she said she'd always text them where she was going instead, and come home when she said she would. And they agreed, because she kept her word and never made her parents wonder where she was and if she was safe.

Acting like an independent adult also means acknowledging that your parents may still have rules in their house that you need to follow even if you no longer live there full time. For example, Kim Cook didn't allow her college-age daughters to drink in the house when they were under twenty-one, because that's the law. If anything were to happen, she would have been held legally responsible, and so that rule stood even though her daughters may have been drinking at school. Similarly, if you have younger siblings who have to wake up early for school, a really late curfew might not be feasible for you. You may not agree with it, but you should be able to see that it's not unreasonable that your parents want to avoid the door slamming at 2 AM. But one area where you can put your foot down is your sex life. If you find your parents getting just a touch too nosy about your intimate relationships, a simple "I don't see how that's really your concern" should make your boundaries pretty clear. If you want your parents to see you as an adult, you need to show them you're up to the task of acting like one.

COMMUNICATION 101

Parental Conflict in College

Regardless of the type of relationship you had with your parents beforehand, leaving home for college can really alter the ways you communicate. Perhaps the most notable way that happens? Decontextualization. Dr. Damour explains: When you live at home with your parents, they're with you for all sides of an issue or a conflict. They can see when you get upset about something, maybe they can help talk it out, and they'll see the eventual resolution after The Problem slowly works itself out. They know you're okay because they get to see it with their own eyes. When you're living away at school, they don't have the extra context around a problem that they might glean from being with you. They only have the bits of information you might offer them, which often isn't the full picture, so they don't understand the scope of whatever you're dealing with—especially the part where it eventually gets better. Naturally, they worry! This is compounded by a behavior among adolescents that Damour calls "dumping the emotional trash." Young adults sometimes tell their parents or family about a problem they're experiencing. They feel better having unburdened themselves of something upsetting, and often, these conversations end on a negative note. Your parents are then left with an uncomfortable feeling and they continue to worry without knowing that ten minutes after you hung up the phone, you started to feel better.

It's not that this is developmentally inappropriate—it's great to start keeping more of your life private and find resolutions on your own—but keep in mind that if you're only sharing negative news with your parents, it's going to freak them out unnecessarily and probably generate conflict. Thankfully, there's a pretty easy workaround: Even if you're calling your parents about something that's annoying you, toss in some-thing positive, like a great lecture you went to last week. Or text them out of the blue if you earned a good grade on a challenging paper. Little things like this will go a long way, especially in the early days of college.

Then of course, there will be the conflicts unique to college that are a bit tougher to tackle. With more autonomy and a bedroom wherein you can admit whoever you please, but still connected to your family through practical things like bank accounts, car leases, and food bills, you might find your back against a wall when things that aren't your parents' business, well, sort of become their business. For example, Kacey's not being able to use her family insurance for her birth control. Because of her off-campus job she could afford to pay out of pocket, but not everyone will have that luxury. If you can, try to approach these conversations in advance before you even leave for school. An expert-approved conversation starter: "Hey, I realize that while I'm in school I'm on your insurance. Thinking ahead, there might be times where I may use that for certain parts of my health, including things related to my sexual health. I want to be able to talk to you openly about these things if I need to. What are your thoughts?" Then it'll be less of a shock to them if something seems amiss with the family deductible.

Raising Tricky Topics

If you need to talk to your parents about an important issue that you think they're unlikely to be super sympathetic toward, Kim Cook sug-gests the buddy system. You know those mentors we mentioned earlier? Grab one you know really well, ideally a family member, and ask them if they'll hop on a phone call to your parents with you. Here is the only thing they need to say to your parents: "Hey, you know, [insert your name] had to [insert issue here: See a doctor, get a test done, access birth control] and I'm here to support her." That's it! They don't even need to speak for the rest of the call. You'll feel like you have someone in your corner during a vulnerable conversation, and your parents may be less likely to overreact if there's someone else on the line.

Other times, simply the nature of your growing independence can cause a row. Take Imogen, a senior at a large city university. Imogen told me about the time she went on a family vacation to visit her sister, who had moved out of state. Before she left for the trip, she'd been messaging with a guy she met on Instagram who lived in the area. They hit it off and planned to meet when she would be in town. A few days into the trip, Imogen told her family she was going out on a date that evening, and she wasn't sure what time she'd be back. She wound up staying out all night. When she got home, her father was furious. According to Imogen, he was annoyed she didn't come home in the evening, but when she explained that she was out all night with a guy, he was livid. He inferred, correctly—from the fact that she didn't come home—that they had had sex, and launched into a tirade of judgmental questions and accusations. He pleaded with Imogen to realize that this guy was using her. He wondered how she could possibly have sex with someone she didn't love. He all but outright called her a whore. None of this made room for the fact that his adult daughter had a consensual sexual experience that both she and her partner enjoyed.

Parents can struggle at this stage, in my experience, because they've run out of realistic punishments and consequences when you do something they don't like. If they're paying for college, for example, they're unlikely to pull you out of school unless your academic performance is truly suffering or your health is in danger. If it weren't, that puts them in a tough position to explain to inquiring relatives why, for example, little Suzie, president of the Student Government Association and a straight-A student, is no longer attending college. ("Well, she was having sex, and I didn't . . . like . . . that?" wouldn't play well at cocktail parties.) If you're paying for your own education or on a scholarship, they have even fewer cards to play. They can't really ground you, because you're an adult. Maybe they can take your car keys, but Uber and Lyft are nearly everywhere. They likely won't confiscate your phone, because then they can't reach you. Imogen's father briefly threatened to send her home from the family vacation early, but that fizzled. Who wants to pay for airline change fees, anyway?

I say this not as carte blanche to go pissing off your parents simply because you're a legal adult, but to help you understand where they're coming from. Feeling powerless is an uncomfortable emotion; it might make you lash out and say things you don't mean in a desperate bid to feel heard and respected. Your parents are human and they are flawed, but that doesn't mean they don't love you. Even if they're wrong about their understanding of and approach to a situation, they're often just trying to keep you safe. I like Imogen's story specifically because it's messy. Do I think it's totally safe to hook up with a stranger you met on an app without taking a few dates to get to know them? Not really. Have I done it myself? Ask my last Tinder date.

Imogen isn't blithely unaware of the risks. She's a good student who holds down an internship and a part-time job at school. And while I want to reiterate that no amount of responsibility on your end can prevent an assault from someone who wants to harm you, Imogen did try and plan ahead. Imogen asked her sister in advance about a good, safe spot for a date, and her sister suggested a bar where she knew the owner. Then, her sister got in touch with the owner and asked him to look out for her little sister, just to be safe. (It's always a good idea to let people know where you're going on a first date; better still if there will be people you know there!) She also circulated his social profiles with her friends and sister so people would know who he was and what he looked like. Then, she spent a few hours with him at the bar getting to know him better before they went home together. Is this foolproof? Not a bit. Someone can harm you no matter how nice they seem, whether it's a day or a month into a relationship. But it does show foresight on her part that maybe would have comforted her father to know.

Dr. Damour agrees that both Imogen and her father could have approached things differently. While Imogen's dad struggled to accept his daughter is an adult sexual being with active desires, he also had some legitimate safety concerns. Damour suggests he might have been better off saying something like, "I trust that you did something you wanted to do. But I wouldn't be much of a parent if I didn't express my concern that this doesn't sound all that safe to me. Could you help me sleep better at night by explaining to me how you knew it was safe or what you did to make sure it was safe?" Then, they might have had an opening to talk more about what's required for truly consensual sex: communication, trust, and a feeling of safety. It can be hard to really enjoy sex if you're worried about safety, even if it's just a fleeting thought in the back of your mind. He could have asked if she really had enough of a relationship with this guy to talk openly about what they both wanted? All of those would have been better places to start a conversation than by attacking her motivations and actions. Not many parents have the foresight to ask thoughtful questions like these when they're agitated, but you can do your best to steer the conversation without getting worked up. Try something like, "Hey, have you thought about asking me XYZ? I might have an answer you'd like to hear."

For her part, Imogen probably shouldn't have stayed out all night without a follow-up text letting her family know so that her dad wasn't worrying all night. She also could have preemptively shared some of the steps she took to have a safer encounter so that the conversation was less about her sex life and more about general common sense and finding common ground. Your parents just want to know you're safe and not lying in a ditch somewhere, no matter how old you are.

COMMUNICATION 201

Staying in Touch without Going Insane

One of the biggest points of contention that I had with my parents when I was in college was about my habit of calling home, or lack thereof. It's not that I didn't want to talk to them, I just didn't want to stop what I was doing and talk on the phone for an extended amount of time. There's a difference! And for good reason, too. Especially in the early days of college, you're trying to make friends, learning where the academic buildings are, making Target runs when you realize there are so many things you forgot to pack, and maybe awkwardly hooking up with some of the guys who live on your dorm floor. We'd schedule calls and then I'd keep missing the appointment. There are honestly not enough hours in the day for hours-long catch-up calls, but that doesn't mean you have free rein to ignore your parents. Here's what you (and your parents) can do instead.

1. Embrace "drive-bys."

A phenomenon shared with Damour by a fellow parenting expert, drive-bys in this context mean short visits from parents. Parents weekend is really fun, until it's been seventy-two hours straight of Mom and Dad and you want to hang out with your friends instead. So, parents, keep visits brief—like swooping into town on a business trip and taking your kids and their friends out for dinner, then leaving. Or coming in to see a sports match on campus, and then a quick lunch. This way, it's an exciting event to look forward to, but you have the promise that it won't last forever, and you won't be awkwardly stuck trying to make your parents fit into your college social life.

2. Don't just call, write.

Embrace text messages and email for tiny missives throughout the week, just to show your parents you're alive and thinking of them. And parents, vice versa! Something like, "Saw these shoes, thought of you." Or, "Let's make this recipe when I'm home next break," sends a message you're on each other's mind. Plus, notes like the latter that are future-thinking will convey that you're looking forward to spending time together even when you're apart. You can have a text convo back and forth, of course, but what's great about a quick note is that it doesn't necessarily demand an immediate response from either party, which matters during the busy college years.

3. Give yourself something to talk about.

If you have trouble sticking to scheduled phone calls or find yourself running out of things to say, Kim Cook suggests getting intentional and creative with how you stay in touch. At the beginning of the semester, you can share your course reading list with your parents. If you have any common interests, you can both pick one book to read in tandem so you'll have something specific to touch base about. This can encourage the types of conversations where you both respectfully share opinions, which can help solidify your parents' view of you as a more independent adult. Another creative tactic Cook suggests to get the conversation gears moving? Parents, Venmo your kid five or ten bucks every now and then and ask them to send you a picture of what they spent it on. (And please think carefully about just how honest you want that photo to be!)

Whatever methods of communication you think will work best for you, talk to each other in advance about how often, and in which ways, you'll reach out when you're at school. If you can agree on expectations beforehand, it's less likely to cause a fight.

Feeling Clingy? Homesick?

For many, your parents and family might be the bedrock of your life, the people who make you feel safe and accept you for who you are. It's normal that going away to college might not be the carefree opportunity it is for some to stretch their wings, but instead a lonely transition accented with homesickness and growing pains. While calling your parents all the time or heading home every weekend might feel tempting, it can prevent you from getting settled at school and making friends. Here are expert-approved strategies to tackle that wistful nostalgia that might creep in during the first semester, or maybe even beyond.

1. Take a step back and realize that whatever you're feeling is okay.

Think about how much extra work your brain has to do in a new environment. You have to figure out a new system (be it card, or keys) to get into your room. You have to keep track of where each new classroom is in each new hall in each new building. You have to calculate how long it takes to walk or drive from your dorm so you're not late for class. You have to figure out the best times in your schedule to squeeze in meals, and start to build up some friends to eat with. You have to get to know your peers and get a sense of what clubs are out there, and if you'd like to join any. You have to figure out which of the clothes dryers leave your laundry soaking wet and which actually work. There are parties, fights with roommates, first hookups, and so much more. The mental work you're doing to make sense of it all is *exhausting*. It makes sense that you'd miss home, where you already know how everything works and your parents are right there to fix your laundry mishaps. Conventional wisdom says it can take up to a full year to get truly settled in new surroundings, so start by reminding yourself that it's too early to have anything figured out. This is natural!

2. Give yourself emotional goals.

When everything seems hard and you're missing home, force yourself to find something to be excited about. Is there a dance performance you want to go see? A date? A splurgy meal off-campus with a friend? Put these things, every single one, on your calendar. Mapping out these fun, distracting activities will give you something to look forward to all the time. Bonus: While you're doing them, you may eventually start to feel more and more connected to your new home away from home and all it has to offer.

3. Be aware of your backup options.

There's a chance your homesickness is just that, but it could also be your brain's way of telling you this school just isn't the right fit. When I called home telling my parents how much I hated college and my school, they told me, well, you can always transfer. Which might be true for you, too! You could defer a year, try a school closer to home, or even take your education totally online. If these sound like options you may want to take, get a sense of when the deadlines are to send in those transfer applications and what materials you'll need from your current school early, just in case. I absolutely wound up loving my college by my second semester, but just hearing that I didn't have to stay and knowing the practical steps I'd need to take to try something new really helped me relax.

4. Keep an eye on your communication patterns.

If you go running to your high school friends and parents for everything that goes wrong in college, you're losing the chance to build support networks where you are now who genuinely want to be there for you. If you're someone who feels overly reliant on your community from home, try to think of communication like lines on a graph. As time goes by, try to see your calls home decreasing and your reliance on new friends at school increasing. I really hate math, but even I can handle this one.

College is, without a doubt, a time of change. Some you might expect, others will be completely surprising. Some your family will embrace, others they might feel unprepared for. But with an open mind and this guide, you can face them head-on.

ℓℓℓℓ

After repeatedly encouraging you to cut your parents some slack and try to understand their point of view even if you don't agree with it, what kind of hypocrite would I be if I didn't even try, some fifteen years later, to do the same? I called up my mom and, one by one, asked her about the events that shaped my understanding of sex the way *she* saw them. To the birth control debacle, she acknowledges, "That sounds like something I would say." To the panicked phone calls after my visit with the school nurses, she stood firm: "I think everyone should be discerning when it comes to who you sleep with." Well, fine.

But our conversation about the trip with my boyfriend surprised me in both its honesty and nuance. I'm the youngest of two daughters, which is to say, I'm my parents' baby—even in my thirties. Perhaps related to my mom's desire to keep me in a state of perpetual infancy, she wasn't ready for her youngest child to be having sex. In fact, she remembers me as being much younger than the seventeen years I was when we had that fight. And more than that, she felt like she'd somehow failed me as a parent, like she let me go into an unsupervised situation and felt misled when she started to realize that maybe my boyfriend and I weren't just holding hands (even though we both acknowledged I hadn't done anything wrong). I was confused and hurt at the time, but I hadn't accounted for the fact that my mom might have been angry and disappointed with herself, and not me. Those are powerful emotions that can cloud your ability to see others clearly. When I came home after the vacation, she explained, she just didn't know how to talk about it. So instead my mom adopted a "what's done is done" attitude.

I'll go out on a limb here and say that the relationship between mother and daughter may be the most complex you'll ever have. In that regard, do I feel like I got the short end of the stick when it comes to sex and feelings of internalized shame and rejection? Yes. But in my house, my mom was also the one who could fix anything. Doctor appointments were instantly scheduled at the first sign of malaise, carpools for after-school activities coordinated with ease, essays for English class copy edited handily. My mom made things happen, and she truly wanted us to know we'd have her support no matter what we pursued in life. Even my dad, who never took a starring role in the birds-and-bees portion of my upbringing (shocking, I know) surprised me as a teenager by ensuring I heard one message loud and clear: Make sure you're never beholden to a man for anything. He wanted to be certain I could rely on myself. That I'd never be too scared to leave a bad relationship because my partner paid the rent. That I'd always have a career and skills of my own that no one could take away. Progressive-ish!

All this to say, no matter where your family falls short, there are probably areas of your care at which they excel. Let them know when you need more from them, but try and celebrate your wins now, too. You don't have to wait fifteen years to acknowledge all they do for you, like someone else I know.

10.

The Gray Areas

How to Recognize Sexual Assault That Doesn't Always Look Like Assault

> Heads-up: This chapter contains frank conversations about sexual assault. If this will be too hard for you to read, but you're interested in strategies for healing after assault, skip to page 228.

Not long after I graduated college, I ran into a guy I vaguely knew at a party. "Ran into," in this case, being code for "took one look at this person and decided that the night would be a complete and utter failure if I did not have sex with him." So I made my interests known: sustained gazes in his direction and then shyly darting my eyes away, sneaking dirty double entendres into group conversations hoping he'd laugh, announcing that I'd be heading into the other room to mix a new drink to see if he'd follow (he did). Does my flirting sound aggressively corny in retrospect? Sure, but at that time in my life it typically got the job done, so I wasn't ready to overhaul the system just yet. We left the party together and went back to his apartment, where we had another drink. Then what usually happens (when two people who have been hot for each other all night finally get away from the crowd) happened: We had sex. Given that this night was nearly ten years ago, the memory is fuzzy to me now, made more so by the booze. I remember how crazy it felt that someone this stupidly attractive was into me, I remember really wanting to sleep with him, I remember enjoying it, and I remember we used a condom. We reclothed ourselves, pink-cheeked and giggly, and adjourned to the living room, where we split a joint. And, naturally, having the libido of early twentysomethings, we quickly found ourselves scrambling back to the bedroom to have sex again.

When we were done, I realized that the second time around, he hadn't worn a condom. I was a little stoned, a little buzzed, and very confused. We had used one the first time at my request; why would this time have been different? I asked him about it, to which he replied, "You didn't say anything, so I figured it was fine." And when he added, "How could you not have realized? Did you think it was just some sort of magical, skin-textured condom?" I was all but humiliated into dropping the subject. He thought he was making a hilarious joke about something that was no big deal ("Ha ha! A condom that feels like a naked dick!") But I was left playing catch-up, trying to figure out why I felt so vulnerable and betrayed. The sex itself was consensual, enthusiastically so, which made it even harder to parse out what, exactly, felt so wrong. After we both discussed some recent STI test results, I shrugged it off. No harm done, I reasoned. I went on to hook up with him for a few more months.

But there *is* harm done when someone changes the criteria of what you consented to and just hopes you won't notice. It's sexual misconduct at a minimum, and depending on the circumstance, sexual assault. These moments, especially the ones that exist in a murky gray area of our minds, can be hard to process. If someone attacks you in a dark alley you'd instantly know it's wrong; you'd feel entitled to your rage and your grief. But when you all but begged to get naked with someone and then suddenly something just feels off? That's more complicated to cope with. You're left with the guilt: *I shouldn't have been drinking, I shouldn't have been smoking.* The confusion: *Maybe he did ask me, and I just forgot.* The embarrassment: *I feel like an idiot, I don't want him to know this bothered me, I want to keep things chill.*

No matter what feelings you're still processing in the wake of an assault, helplessness and loneliness don't have to be among them. Here, you'll hear from other women who've been through it, learn what to know about your campus resources, and get expert guidance on how the healing process begins.

ℓℓℓℓ

Sexual assault is prevalent on college campuses, and the experts I spoke to agree that the years just after high school present the highest risk for assault.[1] The standard statistics say about 1 in 5 women in college will experience sexual assault.[2] However, a more recent survey suggests that the prevalence is higher, pegging it at about 1 in 4 undergrads.[3] Then, think about all the reasons you might not disclose an assault, even to a survey or well-meaning researcher. You're ashamed. You don't like thinking or talking about it. You don't know whether the data collection is truly anonymous. You're not even sure what happened to you "counts" as sexual assault. Bundle all of those together, and it's possible that the statistics are even higher.

We know there's a huge problem, but we don't all experience violence equally. While trans, nonbinary, and genderqueer students are thought to experience similar rates of sexual assault as straight cisgender women do, they experience higher rates of harassment, stalking, and intimate partner violence.[4] We also know that Native American women experience a higher rate of sexual assault compared to people from other groups.[5]

The numbers matter. We can use them to track improvement and to help identify useful interventions. They help you understand and believe that you're not alone. But when it's happening to you, the last thing you care about are the statistics.

First Things First: What Is Title IX and Why Should You Care?

Real talk: I had no idea what the hell Title IX was by the time I got to college. Maybe it was a failure of the American school system, maybe I was more interested in picking out the pattern of my bedspread for my dorm room, who knows? Long story short, Title IX is a civil rights law in the United States that prohibits sex-based discrimination in education, and it's your strongest legal protection when it comes to sexual assault and harassment at school. How does that work? Enter Alexandra Brodsky, a civil rights attorney. She explains courts have recognized that sexual harassment can seriously interfere with a student's education. If a school fails to address that sexual harassment, then the school might be liable for sex discrimination.

There are a few measures your school needs to take to remain compliant with Title IX, like publicly listing a nondiscrimination notice, but the requirement that will likely matter most to you from a practical standpoint is having a Title IX Coordinator. Your school is required to publicly list the coordinator's name and contact info, and my first official bit of advice on this subject is to learn it, even before you get to campus freshman year. In many cases, the coordinator is the person to whom you would report a sexual assault or from whom you would request accommodations in the wake of an assault. My sincerest hope is that you will not need to use this information in your four years of college, but if you can take one logistical hurdle off your plate during a time of great stress, why wouldn't you? If you could be the person to swoop in with all the necessary details for a friend in need, why wouldn't you? Learn about your resources in advance, and it'll be one less task for you to do if you ever need to use them.

In that spirit, here's a bit of what you might be able to expect if you decide to report sexual assault or harassment at school.

HOW THE REPORTING PROCESS WORKS

While at some schools you may be able to tell a trusted professor about what happened, at others you'll need to speak with the Title IX Coordinator directly in order to trigger the school's responsibilities, so start there. After that, the proceedings may vary. A particularly well-resourced school, Brodsky explains, might have trained investigators who will do an initial review and write up their findings. At smaller or less-well-resourced schools, it may be a dean who conducts some initial interviews. The next step would be the hearing, which can either look quite formal or be more like a conversation. You may expect professors or deans to be present as a decision-making panel. Even though school proceedings have become more formal and adversarial over the years, Brodsky adds, no matter what, they're not going to look like the intense trials you see on TV courtroom dramas. The panel will then take interviews and any evidence under consideration and come to a decision. If sanctions are appropriate, the panel will decide those, too.

A quick note here on "evidence." If you're left wondering, *How can I possibly prove what happened to me actually happened?*, don't let that alone stop you from reporting. "A survivor's word is evidence," Brodsky says. "You're not required to have any more to come forward." That said, it's likely you have a lot more support for your report than you think you do. Oftentimes, Brodsky explains, a dormmate down the hall or next door may have heard something. Or you may have texts from the person who assaulted you. If they sensed you were upset, they might have sent you a half-assed apology like, "Sorry things got a little crazy last night." Even friends noticing that you withdrew after the incident might lend indirect support to your claims, Brodsky adds. Bottom line: If you want to report, your word is all you need.

WHAT MIGHT COME AFTER

If your school decides that someone has committed sexual assault, be they staff member or student, there is a range of possible outcomes and sanctions. On the furthest end of the spectrum could be expulsion, termination, or suspension. A less severe outcome might be removal from a class you're in or having their dorm moved. Your school might also put safety plans in place to make sure you don't run into them on campus, like setting up a schedule for when they're allowed to be in communal buildings like the dining hall, let's say. Or mandating certain paths to take between classes to avoid contact. These decisions are often made, Brodsky says, based on how much of a threat the school deems the offender to be toward the rest of the student body, but also based on what you need to have a safe environment in which to learn.

THERE ARE RESOURCES AVAILABLE EVEN IF YOU DON'T WANT TO REPORT

Even if you don't want to go through the formal reporting process, or even if the school doesn't rule in your favor, there are still plenty of accommodations at your disposal that could make a world of difference following the trauma of an assault. For one, your school can allow you to retake a test or even a class if you were having difficulty focusing or studying after the incident occurred. They can also provide tutoring to help catch you up if you've missed classes, or offer an extension on a paper you were unable to turn in. They can also connect you with mental health services. The point being, there are some robust accommodations that your school can offer under Title IX to help you fulfill the most important task of attending school: being a student. To access these services without opening up an official report and investigation, Brodsky suggests approaching your Title IX Coordinator or a confidential mental health provider. It's also important to note that if you did report, these proceedings can sometimes drag out for months. You're entitled to ask for what's called interim accommodations while the proceedings are ongoing, even before they reach a decision. It wouldn't be unreasonable to ask that the offender be prevented from entering your dorm building during this time, for example.

TO REPORT OR NOT TO REPORT?

There usually aren't strict requirements that you have to report immediately, Brodsky explains. If you feel like you might like to lodge a complaint in the future, but not yet, you might talk to your Title IX Coordinator to learn more about the school's policies, and how you might create a record of your experience that could help you in the future. Let's say you're not in a place emotionally to file a report, but you're worried that person might assault someone else. In some rare cases, you may even be allowed to say, "Hey, I don't want to file a formal report right now, but can I be alerted if anyone else files a report against this particular individual?" Like all the accommodations discussed here, your school isn't required to grant you everything you ask for, but knowing your rights under Title IX and asking for what you need is the best way to advocate for yourself.

You have a right to report your assault and seek accommodations, but that doesn't mean you *have* to. My hope in explaining this process is that if you know what to expect, the course of events that follow will perhaps be less overwhelming. We all handle trauma in different ways, and there's no one right way to process an assault. I won't pretend that making a report will be pleasant or easy. The whole ordeal will likely cause you to relive the events that occurred when you share them in interviews. If proceedings don't move quickly, it can make it feel like this agonizing event just never ends, delaying your feeling of closure. The person you're bringing charges against could gossip with their friends and maybe even retaliate against you. Schools can be small communities, and people can be assholes.

Then, of course, there's another big question: How will I feel if the school decides my attacker did nothing wrong? It can be absolutely devastating to feel like no one believes you. If you're having trouble deciding what course to take, Brodsky might ask, "What is going to make you feel like you can continue to learn and stay in school?" If you know you truly cannot continue to share space with them, be it class or campus, you may decide to move forward with reporting. If you want to make sure your academics aren't suffering, you might decide to forgo an official report and explore accommodations on your own. In some cases, your school might be able to facilitate an arrangement where, in lieu of a formal report, the harasser will agree to switch out of a dorm or class themself. But keep your mental health in mind first and foremost. If you know talking about the incident is incredibly difficult and painful for you, to the point where you might be re-traumatizing yourself by going through with a report, don't hesitate to take a step back. Dealing with the assault with the guidance of a therapist and close support systems may be the healthiest choice for you, and that's perfectly okay. And, as Brodsky says, "A school's decision about whether or not they believe something happened doesn't affect whether it actually happened or not."

You may also want to report your assault to the police. While your university likely has systems in place to support you, if you want to press charges, you'll need to file a police report. You don't need to decide if you want to press charges right away, but getting a rape kit exam done ASAP before you shower can help preserve any evidence on your body. If you go ahead with an exam, you can expect to give the provider a medical history, undress, and have swabs taken from your genitalia, fingernails, and mouth to collect any DNA from your assaulter.[6]

Rosemary, a senior at a small school in the Pacific Northwest, made the choice not to report a rape that occurred her sophomore year. Rosemary had just gotten out of a relationship, and her ex-girlfriend was the one Rosemary would typically go to parties with. So, as she prepped for a night out, she started texting people to meet up. She took a shot or two and left. By the time she got to the party, though, all of the people who had agreed to hang were way drunker than she expected. She remembers a lot of men were there, and it seemed pretty rowdy. But she knew the girl who lived in the house and was hosting the party, and felt comfortable enough to stay. Throughout the night, she lost track of her friends. Rosemary recalls one guy repeatedly approaching her, but she consistently brushed off his advances. Eventually, she realized she was too drunk to go home and didn't think it was safe to walk back to her dorm in the middle of the night. The host of the party set up a blanket on the couch, put a glass of water next to her, and they all called it a night. The next thing Rosemary remembers was a man shining his phone's light in her face and telling her, "You shouldn't be on the couch, you should be in bed, come on." At the time, Rosemary was still drunk and hazy from being woken from a deep sleep. She didn't register who was talking to her or what was happening. She followed him into one of the house's bedrooms. Rosemary doesn't have a lot of memories of what happened next, although she's been working with her therapist and understands it's normal to have recollections of sensations but not necessarily chronological events. She remembers the feeling of a beard on her face. She remembers him smelling of beer. Her next concrete memory is waking up an hour later, very sober and very disoriented. She was naked (and she never slept naked), and a man's hand was across her. She saw a used condom on the floor. Rosemary gathered her things, left the room, chugged her water from the night before, and left.

Later that morning, one of her friends called her to chat. They were talking about how their nights went, and when she explained the strange scene she woke up to, he told her it sounded pretty shady. "And then it kind of hit me. I just felt really, really terrible," Rosemary says. She never told her friend who was hosting the party, and she never tried to figure out who the man who raped her was. "My initial feeling was shame. And embarrassment. Like, my mom taught me better than that. I should— that should not have happened . . ." she says, trailing off. "And then I just wanted to forget it." Her friend on the phone tried to convince her to report it, but Rosemary had just served as a juror for a sexual assault case in court. She watched a case between two students that was similar to what she experienced play out in front of a judge, and the guy involved didn't get convicted on any charges, not even a misdemeanor. "I saw how emotional she was and I just did not want that for me," Rosemary says. The consensus she came to was, why bother? It's worth noting that campus proceedings are generally less intense and invasive than going to trial in court, but I understand her mindset. She was also afraid of letting the event define her, and being known as the girl who got drunk at a party and got raped. Now, though, Rosemary is doing better. She's working with her therapist, accepting care from the people who love her, and reminding herself that no matter what happened, it wasn't her fault. She told me she wished she could have been braver and reported it, but at the time she just wanted to focus on taking care of herself. I didn't say it at the time, but I think taking care of herself is the bravest thing she could have done.

RECOGNIZING IT'S WRONG 101
Not All Abuse Feels Like Assault

It's unfathomably easy to think we know what all abuse will look and feel like, or to assume we know how we might react. The reality is that violence and harassment exist on such a wide spectrum that the spectrum itself can blind us to what's going on, or shape our reaction to it. We tend to think if something wasn't what we typically think of as violence ("I said 'no' and he forced himself on me anyway" or "He hit me until I agreed to have sex") then it's not a big deal. And that feeling of "other people have it worse" can often cause us to brush off what were very real harms done to us. Sometimes you're not even sure that what happened was assault in the first place until months or years later.

Piper recently graduated from Stanford University. She was active in student life, including organizations that ran feminist-centered programming on campus. But even being tuned in to issues women face in their intimate relationships, she wasn't immediately able to categorize what happened to her one night as assault. Piper's friend's boyfriend had a friend who wanted to be set up with her, and she agreed to take him as her date to a dinner event being hosted on campus. They had what she describes as a lovely night with great conversation, and as they headed to another party at his frat, she knew this was someone she wanted to hook up with. She felt confident enough in their chemistry that she knew she wanted to have intercourse, specifically. "In my head,

I decided that for myself and was like, *This feels fine. If that's where the night goes, I feel good about that,*" she explains. And it did go there. At this point in the night they were both drunk and went back to his dorm room together.

Piper had recently gotten out of a long-term relationship, and although she'd been having some casual sex, she always used protection—which is likely why she remembers asking the guy if he had a condom. He didn't have one, but insisted they could still have sex. Piper kept saying no, and he kept trying to persuade her otherwise. She remembers him coaxing her, saying that they were both "clean," so it was fine. Piper specifically remembers being disgusted and objectified by that phrasing. (And for good reason. Not only is it stigmatizing language, he was implying that the only legitimate reason she might not want to have unprotected sex was because of STIs, completely ignoring her right to bodily autonomy.) He kept trying, performing oral sex on her, and doing whatever he could to get her in the mood.

Although she doesn't have an exact timeline of the events, at some point she recalls that he started having sex with her, even though at no point did she indicate she wanted to. He tried to wear her down, and when that failed, figured he'd go for it anyway. She described the idea of getting up to leave as "impossible." She had just had so little experience shutting down something once it already started, she explains. I don't have to tell you that this is a clear example of nonconsensual sex. But that didn't register to Piper right away. She recalls cataloging it in her head with the nebulous term "bad sex," and repressing the experience. Except trauma doesn't always go away quietly.

Not long after, Piper entered a phase she describes as "being very reckless with [her] body," drinking more than usual and having unprotected sex, including ensuing pregnancy and STI scares. It wasn't until a year later, at the start of the #MeToo movement, that an image shared on Facebook made her reframe what happened to her as assault.

Suddenly, Piper started to understand the choices she had recently been making more clearly. When someone doesn't treat your boundaries with care, it can sometimes make you feel like your body isn't worthy of care at all. Compounding her initial hesitancy were headlines about the widely reported trial involving Brock Turner and Chanel Miller, a cut-and-dry case of rape on campus that had all but taken over the news. Piper thinks, looking back, that the frenzy surrounding the trial made it harder for her to identify what happened to her as assault, because her experience was so dissimilar. After all, she knew this guy. She liked him. She wanted to have sex with him. She was drunk, but she wasn't unconscious. "I think that the more extreme you make the definition, the harder it is to put yourself in that definition. It makes it more exclusive," she explains. But even if it took her time to get there, she's given herself the space to see that event for the violation it was. Piper worked with a therapist, and after we spoke, she decided she wanted to contact her school's Title IX office, even though she had graduated, just to have it on record. The school told her that what happened to her could be considered a crime and gave her some resources to pursue legal action. That exchange alone was meaningful for Piper. "It felt like a win. In a world of mostly Ls, it was definitely a win."

To be absolutely clear: Sexual assault is not limited to acts of intercourse. Someone who knows that is Meredith, who came from a small town in the South and attended an all-women's college in New England. After completing a high school education that was entirely online, she was excited and apprehensive about her college experience: being in a new, in-person social environment 24-7. Her upbringing was fairly conservative, with a no-sex-before-marriage mentality. She figured she'd go off to college, find a husband, and that would be that. All this to say, she didn't expect college would be a time when she'd start exploring her attraction to women and get an up-close view of how hookup culture and male entitlement function at school. Meredith was involved with Black student life organizations at her school, and recalls one night attending a multicultural organization party at a neighboring co-ed school. She was dancing and enjoying the party when suddenly she felt someone behind her grab her breasts. Although Meredith wasn't yet sexually active, she understood that there was going to be a certain degree of physical proximity when you're grinding with someone on the

It can be hard to articulate your boundaries if you haven't had much practice communicating about your body.

dance floor. She was fine with that. It's to be expected that your dance partner might have their hands on your waist or hips, or that you might even be positioned butt-to-crotch while you get in the flow of the song. But there's no dance move that involves grabbing someone's breasts, and Meredith instantly felt violated. She says the exchange was probably no longer than a moment, but it felt much longer. "The grime of the experience has stayed. And I know that I thought about that night for a while afterward," she explains. Meredith spent the rest of her college experience avoiding spaces where she'd need to get too close to him. In the moment, though, Meredith just tried to get away to somewhere else on the dance floor. She didn't feel like she was capable of calling him out or telling him to stop, which she attributes to her lack of experience with both sex and dating at the time. It can be hard to articulate your boundaries if you haven't had much practice communicating about your body. Now Meredith is dating someone who she describes as very pro-consent. He puts in the work to talk during sex and make sure she's always on board, which has helped her feel confident communicating about her needs both with him and in general.

RECOGNIZING IT'S WRONG 201
Coercive Control

We've gone over many individual scenarios and sexual encounters, but abuse isn't relegated to one-off nights. Here to shed light on coercive control in relationships is Lisa Aronson Fontes, PhD, senior lecturer II at the University of Massachusetts and expert on coercive control. Coercive control, boiled down, is when one partner controls the other through tactics like humiliation, isolation, and sometimes—but not always—physical violence. If you're thinking, *That sounds pretty fucking scary, but that would probably be easy to spot if it were happening to me,* don't be so sure. Coercive relationships don't always start out that way.

THE RED FLAGS THAT SPELL TROUBLE
1. "Love bombing"
As Fontes explains, this is when early in the relationship, someone showers you with love, attention, and grand gestures. It can feel super romantic at first, but then they might begin to withdraw that affection or give you mixed compliments, leaving you confused, or even desperate, vying to get their attention back. This gives them the upper hand, making you work hard to please them.

2. An all-consuming relationship

The abuser in this scenario might say something like, "Let's drown out the rest of the world and just spend all our time alone together," Fontes explains. That can seem really sweet, in part because we've problematically glamorized an Insta-caption version of relationships ("He's my whole world!").

3. Asking for "proofs" of love

Offering up expressions of love freely, like voluntarily picking up your significant other at the airport, is one thing. You do these things because you want your loved one to know they're cared for. It would feel a lot different if your partner had asked you to chauffeur them around and suggested that if you don't, you must not really love them. Requesting proofs of love can look a lot of different ways, but someone pressuring you into having sex right away could be one. Demanding (or even persistently suggesting) you send nude photos could be another. They may want passwords for your phone or email, or ask you to turn on location sharing "so we can always find each other." But this should ring the alarm bells in your brain. "It can feel wonderful in the beginning," Fontes says. "Like, *Wow, nobody has ever cared that much about me.* It plays into those romantic stereotypes that we might have. But over time, the person who's the target of the coercive control realizes they've lost some of their freedom."

4. Needing to know where you are

Whether it's tracking you on social media or asking your friends if they've seen you lately, the person exerting coercive control may want to keep tabs on you and may start to make you feel like you owe them constant communication of your whereabouts. Just, no.

This is by no means an exclusive list of behaviors that could indicate the beginning of a coercive relationship, but a big underlying theme here is a feeling of being pressured for too much, too soon. Being aware of potential red flags will help you avoid them, but if you find yourself in a controlling relationship, Fontes recommends paying close attention to your personal tech, especially if you've shared any passwords. You should get your computer checked for a keystroke logger (which captures and records what you're typing) before changing all your passwords, to make sure everything is secure and you can't be hacked and tracked. Tell a friend what's going on and enlist as many support systems as you can. Make it very clear to the abuser that you wish to have no more contact with them, and let your university—especially campus police—know, too.

Maybe it seems like I'm fearmongering, but controlling relationships can have severe, lasting impacts on a person. For one, Fontes explains, your self-esteem can really take a hit, due to the likelihood of enduring insults and degradation. It can make it really difficult to trust partners in the future. You might experience sexual trauma, since these relationships can include coerced sex as well. Most relevant to college-specific coercive relationships, however, is the lost time. There's no way to get those months or years back, and the results can be especially damaging because of the decisions you were convinced to make while under someone's influence. You might have dropped out of all your clubs, dropped classes you like to be more available to their scheduling whims. You might have skipped a chance to study abroad, or withdrawn from college altogether. You might have missed out on the chance to make friends. To sum it up, it's a missed opportunity to put yourself first, Fontes explains.

Anyone can be at risk for an abusive relationship—it just takes meeting the wrong person at the wrong time. The risk itself does not belong to you, or anything you did. But being young doesn't always help when it comes to avoiding the red flags right away. The lack of lived experience can make it harder to have that internal barometer we use to compare and assess situations. It's like trying to check if you have a fever without having a thermometer. It makes it harder to say no to bullshit pressures from bullshit guys, because we haven't yet learned that they're bullshit. "If you come to college without experience in relationships, then you don't have as solid a ground to understand what you want and what feels good and what doesn't," Fontes explains. "And if you haven't had the benefit of seeing people around you have healthy relationships, whether it's your parents or neighbors or teachers, then it's hard to know what's the right kind of relationship." That doesn't mean "Go out and have tons of sex before you get to college!!!!!!" But it does mean you should take the time to get to know yourself, your body, and what kinds of qualities you admire in people, even if it's just your friends. That way, you'll have a better idea about what you want—and whether someone is ignoring your wants (big red flag!)—and you'll have the beginning of a framework to compare future relationships to.

> **Take the time to get to know yourself, your body, and what kinds of qualities you admire in people, even if it's just your friends.**

SEXUAL ASSAULT RESISTANCE 101

Practical Tips to Trust Your Gut

I hate the fact that I'm about to share guidance on reducing the likelihood of an assault. I hate that we live in a world where you need this advice. I hate the notion that women feel like it's their responsibility to prevent assault, because it's absolutely not. There's not a single choice you can make that will result in your getting assaulted; the only relevant choice is the one made by the person who decided to assault you. With that said, I'm sharing some practical advice from Charlene Senn, PhD, a professor and a Canada Research Chair in Sexual Violence. I'm sharing it because her program, Flip the Script with EAAA™ (Enhanced Assess, Acknowledge, Act), works. Her program has been proven to significantly reduce both completed and attempted rape in first-year students.[7] The program is divided into four units: Assess, Acknowledge, Act, and Relationships & Sexuality. Because the course is spread out over multiple hours and days, it's impossible to distill everything you'd learn if you took the full course, but there are some incredibly useful nuggets you can start using right away. In no particular order, they are:

1. Think about risk differently.

We've been so conditioned to think about risk for sexual assault as a stranger in a dark parking garage, but that's not even close to the whole picture. You're more likely to be assaulted by someone you know. And yes, the risk of assault is higher when alcohol is present (whether men are drinking, women are drinking, or both). Alcohol gives perpetrators some advantages, Senn notes, but that doesn't make drinking itself risky when it comes to sexual assault. Think about it this way: You could down ten beers, get nearly blackout drunk with your friends, and not get assaulted. That's because the risky part is the presence of a perpetrator. (I do not recommend you drink that much for safety reasons in general, but the point stands!) This can be an incredibly healing shift in mindset. Now let's go back to the parking garage mentality. Isolation is a factor, because perpetrators can have the upper hand without bystanders present, but that isolation can look very different from what you'd expect. Senn urges you to consider factors like sound isolation. For example, if a guy brings you to a different room of a house party, loud music blaring around the corner can act as insulation that isolates you. Or if you're in a multiple-story house and you go upstairs, away from the majority of partygoers. So instead of "stranger in an alley," think "person you've met before who tries to isolate you from the crowd."

2. Look for problematic behavior cues in potential hook-up partners.

It's important to note that everyone can have an off day or snap if they get upset, and that doesn't mean a guy who had a jerk moment once might not be an awesome partner, but stay attuned to these traits and behaviors that could indicate someone more likely to commit assault.

Persistence: Someone who is constantly pressuring you, over and over, in order to get their way—whether it has to do with sex or not—should be a big red flag. This can be over something as simple as what movie you're going to watch that night, and it may even be done with a joking demeanor. Either way, think about the message they're sending you: What I want is more important than what you want.

Sexualizing behavior: The example that Senn gives is of two people meeting for the first time at a party. The guy asks what her major is, and the girl answers, "Biology." He then says, "Good, so you'll know how everything works," with a leering grin. Beware of someone who tries to make everything about sex, or makes things too sexual too quickly. I'm not saying that any guy who makes a dirty joke is a rapist, far from it.

The key here is context. Do they constantly sexualize things? Do they sexualize things right from the jump, before they get to know you? Or do they do it once you've developed a rapport and it's clear that you're both flirting?

Dominance and expressions of anger and hostility: Outbursts of anger and the need to be in control are obviously not great qualities in general, but be on the lookout for those traits especially in regard to how he speaks about other women. If he is constantly saying horrible, inhumane things about his "nasty bitch ex-girlfriend," even if he's sweet as pie to you, that should give you pause. While it's true there are two sides to every breakup, be aware that this could be a marker of how he thinks about women, and how he might talk about and treat you later.

3. Screw being "good."

A large focus of Senn's program has to do with unlearning traditional values you may have been taught. So many of us just want to be good partners, good friends, good people. And that makes it really hard when someone reveals themselves not to have our best interests at heart, because shaking the impulse to smooth things over can be difficult. "For many women, there are all kinds of constraints on what we're supposed to do to make social relationships work better. And when we acknowledge that someone we know is trying to harm us, we need to violate that," says Senn. You are entitled to be loud and to rock the boat when it comes to your boundaries.

4. Fighting back can help.

In the "Act" portion of the program, which is based on Wen-Do Women's Self-Defense, attendees are taught workable self-defense moves in the context of acquaintances. There are no "stranger danger' scenarios taught, to get you more comfortable with the idea of responding physically against someone you know. While self-defense is near impossible to teach in a written format, Senn explained a couple of moves to me. Open your hand with your fingers together, and practice curling each knuckle down until your fingers make a fist as tight as you can get it, with your thumb on the outside. Then strike a target with the fleshy part of your hand nearest your pinkie finger. Practice that on your other palm. See how hard that feels? Senn advises that when you're striking someone, let's say their collarbone, don't just try and make contact. Use maximum power and momentum by beginning with your arm bent at a right angle close to your body. Bring your fist back and around in a circular motion, envisioning yourself striking downward, as though you want to go *through* the collarbone entirely. We're often taught that fighting back will inherently make the situation more dangerous and won't affect the outcome, but Senn says the research doesn't support that, and that physical and verbal resistance can reduce the likelihood of a rape being completed. Another technique is a really loud yell. You want to take a deep breath from your diaphragm (think: belly expanding, not shoulders rising) and yell "Noooooooooooooooooooo!" as loud and as long as you can at a deep register. Senn encouraged me to try it myself, and while I did break into a fit of giggles at the end because it felt so foreign to me, I also completely terrified my dog, so you could say it works! I recommend looking at what classes the National Women's Martial Arts Federation has near you and trying it out for yourself.

5. You deserve to have all the sex you want, and none that you don't.

In the Relationships and Sexuality unit, which comes from Universalist Unitarian Church programming,[8] participants begin to think more critically about their own sexuality and desires. To give you a sense, I'll summarize one exercise called With Whom Would You Do It? that presents various sexual acts, like a blow job or anal sex, and then asks players to decide who they'd feel comfortable doing that act with. Hookup?

Boyfriend? Spouse? Never in a million years? The idea at the heart of it is to start thinking more in-depth about what you actually want. If you haven't considered these questions, it makes it easier for someone to blow past a boundary you didn't know you had. Good sex comes from knowing yourself first. And while these exercises are done without sharing to ensure privacy in Senn's program, you can still give it a shot with a trusted group of your own. The next time you're about to play the same drinking game with your friends for the millionth time in a row, maybe write up a bunch of sex-act note cards and try this instead.

One of the cores of this program is the idea that women should trust their gut. If something feels off to you, it probably is. Don't second-guess yourself into silence because you're worried you misinterpreted something. Don't waste a minute thinking that he didn't actually hear you, or that you might as well get it over with. There's a lot that needs to change about the world to address sexual assault. We need consent education starting at a young age. We need targeted bystander programming to empower others to step in. We need social norms education to hammer home the idea that, no, most men don't support violence against women, and a guy's masculinity would not be called into question if he spoke out. And we need programs like Flip the Script with EAAA™ available everywhere. But until that time, arm yourself with the best information you can get. "The risk of listening to yourself is very low. And the risk of ignoring yourself is very high. You can trust those instincts. The worst thing that happens is that you were wrong, but you're safe," says Senn.

If something feels off to you, it probably is.

AFTER ASSAULT: HEALING 101

It's my most sincere hope that you will never need to do the work of putting yourself back together after a sexual assault. If you do, however, I hope you keep in mind the words of Dr. Anjani Amladi: "The most common myth I see surrounding sexual assault is that 'I'm never going to get better. This is never going to go away. I'm going to feel like this forever.'" This couldn't be further from the truth. Here are some steps on where you might start your healing journey.

1. Therapy

Does it shock you that this is the first item on this list? It shouldn't! Everyone reacts differently to an assault, but the effects can be far-reaching, from your ability to sleep, eat, or focus, to your ability to trust other people. It's critical you get all the support you can, and counselors are trained to gently guide you through some of your worst and scariest thoughts. If you don't have access to mental health services, however, Dr. Amladi explains that even your primary care doctor or ob-gyn could be an unexpected place to seek guidance. "If you're looking for some-body you trust, but not necessarily a therapist, sometimes your doctor will suggest that you check in with them more frequently, like maybe once a month, or once every couple of weeks, especially in the begin-ning to try to help manage the stress and trauma," she adds.

2. Support groups

Sometimes we just can't talk about assault with people who haven't experienced it the same way we can with people who have. That's why sharing insight, progress, and even grief with other survivors can be incredibly healing: There's less pressure to explain yourself, because everyone gets it. Support groups are sometimes formal and lead by therapists, but there are also informal groups of survivors who gather together on their own. They can be online or in person—either way, check them out and broaden your support community.

3. Journaling, yoga, or meditation

These mindful exercises can be very effective at calming the high adrenaline response an assault might provoke, Dr. Amladi explains. Journaling in particular can help you keep track of your triggers: Maybe having your shoulder rubbed or certain sex acts remind you of the initial trauma. Jotting down what's still off-limits can be a useful tactic toward understanding what works for you and what doesn't for future encounters. Yoga and stretching are also strategies to feel more connected with and in control of your body physically, which can be comforting in the wake of an assault. These are also helpful outlets to turn to if you feel yourself wanting to self-medicate with drugs or alcohol. "For some, after something traumatic there's a tendency to want to feel better quickly and just completely numb it out and try to forget that it ever happened. That's the type of behavior that we would like to avoid," Dr. Amladi explains. If you're feeling particularly vulnerable in the time that follows, maybe a boozy rager isn't the best place for you to be, and a night in with Yoga with Adrienne would be better.

How Therapy Works

There are lots of different modalities of therapy—trauma-focused therapy! psychodynamic psychotherapy! supportive therapy!—but the first few sessions are mainly about developing a rapport with each other, Dr. Amladi explains. A good therapist is unlikely to pressure you into sharing before you're ready. The management and processing of a trauma will come later, but not before you've built a relationship. If you don't feel a good vibe with your therapist, you can switch! Just like with dating, it's rare you're going to meet The One right out of the gate.

To get a better sense of what trauma-focused work might look like, here's an example of cognitive behavioral therapy (CBT). Dr. Amladi says to picture a triangle. Each point on a triangle represents a different word: thoughts, feelings, and behaviors. Then if you were to draw double-sided arrows on each side, it becomes easy to visualize that your thoughts can impact your feelings, your feelings can impact your behaviors, your behaviors can impact your thoughts, and so on. CBT focuses on cognitive distortions that can throw that triangle out of whack. If you were a sexual assault survivor, for example, Amladi explains that you might have a cognitive distortion that it was your fault and you provoked it. That thought can impact your behavior, and so on, and make everything spiral out into an anxiety-ridden, guilt-fueled chaos machine. The goal of CBT is to help you reframe those cognitive distortions in a more rational way, which then helps the other points of the triangle.

It's so hard to break the shame-and-guilt cycle of assault because as humans, we often want rational reasons for why something happened, and assault can be incredibly irrational. The exact two people could go to the same party, drink the same amount, talk to the same people, and one might get assaulted while the other gets an Uber home. It's hard to wrap your mind around that. Remember Rosemary, the young woman who didn't want to report her assault? Not long after, she started dating a guy who happened to be at the party that night. He left early, but Rosemary was still holding on to some embarrassment that he might have seen her there and thought she was a mess, and that it was her fault for being drunk. When she ultimately told him about what happened to her, he was sympathetic, but she didn't get the answer she really needed. Her therapist, who Rosemary jokingly calls her "guru," encouraged her to try again. "That took a lot of effort on my part, because I didn't want to risk feeling rejected or feeling like my boyfriend has a bad opinion of me," she says. But she did it anyway, and asked him outright if he thought what happened to her was her fault. And of course, his answer was no. A terrible person did a terrible thing to her. With the encouragement of her therapist, Rosemary was able to start breaking down one of her most irrational thought distortions. A big leap forward on her path to healing.

∾∾∾∾

I still struggle to call what happened to me sexual assault. Would I feel better calling it a consent violation? *Well, I never told him outright I wanted to use protection both times*, I reason with my neurotic self, afraid to claim a label I don't "deserve." Mostly, I'm embarrassed. My intimate life has been all but an open book for the better part of my twenties. I don't leave a lot unsaid because I'm too lazy to hide even my blunders. I figure, at the very least, someone else might learn something from it. Maybe I can make them laugh. Maybe they'll follow me on Twitter. But sharing this particular story left me feeling more vulnerable and humiliated than I'd imagined it would. Like I told the whole world I got tricked into letting a guy take something he wanted, something I didn't want to give.

I'm embarrassed to admit that I still think about him. Sometimes I'll pull up his Instagram, thumb through the photos of his recent comings and goings. It looks like he's doing well. His new girlfriend has a pretty smile. The funny thing is I don't wish him ill at all. I don't feel the need to confront him, to tell him how with just one sentence he degraded me into thinking I had no right to control what happened to my body, that he should get to make whatever decision he wanted. I don't feel the need for anything, really. Just to say that there's no right or wrong way to move on from assault, harassment, or "bad sex." He can take up space in my phone as a reminder of what I used to tolerate, but nowhere else.

11.

Should I Stay or Should I Go?

Breaking Up without Falling Apart and How You'll Know When You've Found Something Special

Here are just some of the incredibly shitty ways I've ended a relationship: by sending a text, by suggesting a "break" when I knew it was actually over, and by slowly withdrawing until the guy in question had no choice but to dump me. All not great. But I'll tell you about the worst thing I have ever done—not to celebrate it, but to own up to it, and in the process hopefully convince you that it's almost always better to take the effort to end a relationship in a humane way. (Yes, I am setting the bar low. Breakups are hard!) I once dated a guy who everyone, my parents included, described as "such a nice boy." And he absolutely was. But I knew from the jump that it wasn't going to work; I just never felt that sexy spark you should feel, especially at the beginning of a new relationship. He was kind, funny, mature, and responsible, but it wasn't clicking. After dating a string of fuck boys, I desperately wanted to see myself with someone like him and didn't have the heart to end it.

The situation came to a head at my birthday party, of all places. In a dark dive bar with music pumping and my boyfriend by my side, I chatted up my friends, took birthday shots, and ate cake. Then, through the door walked one of my exes. The hottest of my exes—and probably the worst one for me emotionally. I had invited him on a whim, back when Facebook events were still a thing and you just checked the box next to the name of everyone you vaguely knew from college and hoped for the best. I assumed he wouldn't come, but secretly hoped he would. And when he sidled up to the bar and asked if he could buy the birthday girl a drink, I felt giddy and guilty all at the same time. At first we were talking, and then we were flirting, his body pressed against mine, and then I didn't care about anyone else in the room, my boyfriend included. Our searing chemistry reminded me of everything lacking in my current relationship. Eventually, after watching me carry out this very public flirtation right in front of him, my boyfriend came up to me and said, "I think I'm gonna go." I don't remember what I could possibly have said to counter that, seeing as how clearly in the wrong I was, but I remember feeling relieved. Relieved that I didn't have to actually break up with him and he'd gotten the message all the same. I wound up leaving my birthday party with a different guy than I'd arrived with.

The next morning, I woke up in my ex's bed with streaky mascara, and sent a text to break things off officially. (Although, like I said, he was smart. I'm pretty sure he'd figured that one out on his own.)

That's when I went from relief to regret; in the bare light of day, the sun streaming into a first-floor-apartment bedroom belonging to a guy who didn't have a top sheet or a headboard, I had to face the fact that what I had done was incredibly cruel. This is the moment I realized I'd forever and deservedly be the worst ex someone ever had, a title you never want to claim. I sat, scanning the floor for my dress, and processed what that would mean. His friends and family would hear the story and hate me forever. *He* would hate me forever. And they would all be well justified. I caused a really good person what I can only guess was a great deal of pain because I was too immature and impetuous to own up to my feelings and level with him honestly when it wasn't working out. I didn't want to be the evil villain by ending it. Turns out, I wound up making myself the evil villain skank whore who cheated on her boyfriend with her ex at her own birthday party! I tried to email him an apology some weeks later and was swiftly rebuffed. I didn't deserve his forgiveness then, and still don't today. The whole ordeal forced me to confront a nasty side of myself, and since I can't go back and change what I did, I've decided to be grateful for what it showed me. We all have the capacity to act selfishly in our relationships, but we have the space for empathy and humanity, too. I never ended a relationship quite so poorly ever again.

COLLEGE BREAKUPS 101

Getting Dumped

Breakups in college are painfully unique, because when you are dating a classmate and the relationship ends you've got nowhere to run. It's normal if you feel like running. No one, perhaps, knows this better than Blake, a recent grad who went to school in Georgia. Blake had several breakups that tested the limits of what one co-ed can handle. Early on in her freshman year, (like, the very first day!) Blake noticed that the guy who lived across the hall was into her. He offered to walk with her around campus, get her food at the dining hall, and so on. She wasn't sure about him at first, but after a couple months of his near-constant flirting, they slept together. Just two days later, after she was finally invested, he told her he wasn't looking for a relationship. It threw Blake for a loop. She remembers running to tell her roommate about his sudden bait and switch, to which her roommate replied that he'd probably come around. Well, he did come around. But he brought another girl with him when he did. Blake explained that the doors in her dorm were heavy and loud. You could hear them whenever someone came and went. So when she heard a familiar hall door open, she ran to her peephole to stake out the situation. That's when she saw him heading into his room with one of her sorority sisters. It's hard to pretend that doesn't sting, especially when you get a Facebook message the next day from the sister in question that reads, "Hey girl, hope there's no hard feelings!!"

What followed was a sudden mix of confusion, jealousy, and desire that sparked an on-again, off-again hookup between Blake and her hallmate, peppered with periods of silence between them. And the proximity that put him and his parade of other dates on immediate display didn't help, either. "The whole time I was wondering, 'Do I like him, or am I just jealous? Do I just not want him giving attention to other people?' The emotions were very muddled," Blake explains, adding that if they hadn't lived so close she probably would have moved on more quickly. But she didn't. She recalls a devastatingly sloppy night, New Year's Eve maybe, when she came home from a party drunk and was locked out of her dorm. Sometime around two o'clock in the morning it seemed like a great idea to bang on his door relentlessly until he opened it, at which point she melodramatically wailed, "I just want to know why you don't love me?" He suggested she go to bed. Looking back, Blake feels like she made a fool of herself, but she's not entirely to blame: The unique setup of college often allows us to act on our worst instincts. As it turns out, it's better not to have immediate access to the room of your ex-hookup! She knows she was only eighteen at the time, but still wishes she had broken things off more cleanly instead of letting the hookup and hurt feelings linger.

Jessica Moloney, a licensed mental health counselor in New York, gets that breakups suck no matter how you slice it, and being in college can intensify the feelings and muck up the logistics. But having handy tools to turn to can make it more manageable.

1. Wallow a little.

Moloney explains that no matter how hard it is, we have to sit in our emotions and let ourselves be upset. Don't get hung up on whether your feelings are justified even if it was just a short hookup that ended. "This is very much a process of grief; it's a major transition no matter how long you were with the person," Moloney says. So screw the pity party and throw yourself what I like to call a Pleasure Party. Surround yourself with every single comfort you can think of. Envelop yourself in your softest, butteriest sweatpants, queue up your favorite feel-good movies, and order your favorite takeout. Intentionally creating a soft nest of comforts where you can lick your wounds will give you the space to feel bummed while cushioning the blow. Just remember not to isolate yourself from friends, Moloney adds.

2. Give the wallowing an expiration date.

You can't stay at the Pleasure Party forever, unfortunately. Moloney explains that when you sit and stew over a relationship for too long, those thoughts can morph into something unhealthy that doesn't reflect the reality of what actually happened. "When we break up with somebody, we tend to glorify relationships, and we remember all the good times and all the good things. But we have to be mindful that that's not everything and there were probably a lot of other things that went into this relationship." If you wallow too long, you can start worrying that this breakup was somehow all your fault, and that you're never going to find someone else again, and all other manner of totally untrue thoughts. There's no magic cutoff for when you're suddenly going to be "over it," but try limiting yourself to just a weekend or two of the really heavy-duty moping.

3. Find ways to channel the energy.
You might still be feeling sad. You might be angry. You might be jealous, or resentful, or wounded, or any number of emotions that can stick inside your chest and make you feel like you're going to explode and implode all at the same time. So Moloney suggests doing something with them. Exercise may work for you: An explosive run or lifting weights at the gym can flood your system with endorphins and clear your head. But if you have a history with eating disorders, or you just don't like exercise, that may not be the wisest choice. You can also try journaling, and there are a few ways to do it. One strategy is just to get out all your thoughts, stream-of-consciousness style. No rhyme or reason, just write about what happened and how you feel to get the thoughts out of your head and onto paper. Another approach, says Moloney, is to be more methodical about it. For example, try writing down each worry you have with a corresponding, rational thought that brings you back to reality. Like, "I feel devastated this relationship is over, but I know it won't be my only one." Or, "I feel really lonely right now, but I know I'm not actually alone because I have family and friends who care about me." Experiment with an energy-channeling strategy that works for you.

A Note on That First Sighting

Especially if you were the one who got dumped, the moment you bump into them for the first time after a breakup can feel daunting. Like, heart in your esophagus, want to throw up and faint simultaneously, daunting. That's normal. While you want to avoid James Bond–level jumping through hoops to avoid them (if you find yourself trying to leave a room through a window or a back door, you've got a problem), it's okay to admit you want to intentionally pump up your self-esteem. Wear your favorite outfit, travel in groups with your friends for support, and straighten your shoulders and pick up your chin. Use body language to fake it till you make it. And don't feel bad about wanting to look good—whatever that means to you—the first time you see an ex. It doesn't make you a bad feminist to want your hair to look the way you like it to or to be in jeans that fit perfectly, or whatever else from your wardrobe spells confidence to you. One strategy that helped me was to come up with one "normal" thing I knew I could say to an ex, because it was important to me to telegraph that I was comfortable enough to chat with them and not cower in a corner. Something like, "Oh I saw that show your band did, that was great," or "Ugh, that test was awful, how do you think you did?" And then after the briefest of smiling exchanges, I'd walk away. The message being, "I am fine and normal but I'm not here to hang on your every word. Just being polite, thanks and goodbye!" Then again, a guy I dated who dropped out of school came back to visit, and I was so nervous that my nonchalant elbow-on-a-table move knocked over an entire tray of drinks at a party. So. Your mileage may vary.

Moloney explains that this "first time" boils down to exposure therapy. After you get through it once, you know it didn't kill you, and that you can do it again.

eeee

COLLEGE BREAKUPS 201

Breaking It Off

As painful as getting broken up with can be, at least there's no stress of a decision to make. It happens, and you deal with it. When you're the one ending things, deciding what to do can bring its own mental anguish. There are a lot of ways to unintentionally make it harder than it needs to be. Case in point, Evelyn, twenty-two, a recent grad who went to school in Ontario, had a little issue with her timing. During her senior year, she broke up with her boyfriend of three years . . . on Valentine's Day . . . right before giving a major seminar presentation. "I went into it and I honestly looked like I'd been punched in both eyes. It was really kind of funny. But I did this presentation on anti-oppressive social work practice and I did really well. Maybe because the professor felt bad for me," Evelyn muses. When push came to shove, Evelyn knew she was about to enter a rigorous postgrad social work program and felt she needed to prioritize her career over her relationship. But yes, she does regret how she handled the breakup—it wasn't just about the bad timing either. Evelyn admitted she's been meeting up with her ex to walk his dog, who she became quite attached to during their relationship, even though this can make it a lot harder to get the space she needs. "It was my first breakup," she says. "That shit doesn't come with a manual, you know?" Fair enough.

How to Make Breakups Less Brutal

From way too much personal experience, here are some general guidelines to ensure your breakup doesn't end with you sobbing through a social work presentation.

1. Be direct.

Sometimes you can't totally articulate why a relationship isn't working anymore, and that's fine. You don't owe your partner a laundry list of reasons it's over—your gut intuition is enough. But that doesn't mean you want to be wishy-washy or suggest going on a break if you know there's no foreseeable future when you'd want to be naked with this person again. That only gives them false hope. If you need a place to start, Moloney suggests some tried-and-true scripts like, "I don't think we fit together as a couple anymore," or "I see us growing in different directions right now." Try to avoid being ambiguous about what you want so the other person doesn't have space to argue and shake your confidence.

2. Be kind.

Consider their feelings, not as a deterrent to your decision, but as a factor in your delivery. So yeah, maybe don't have this conversation on Christmas morning, or the day before their birthday, or during their final exams, or any other number of emotionally significant occasions. Ask yourself the question, "How can I make this not worse for both of us?" Personally, I don't care for additions like, "I love you so much, but . . ." even though it's likely true. It leaves too much space for someone to ask, "Well, if we love each other, can't we work it out?" I'd opt for, "I have a lot of respect for you," or "I really value the time we've had together" as a kind way to gently massage their self-esteem as you tell them you want to end the relationship. Love is a loaded word in the context of a breakup, so use it carefully.

> ### 3. Believe it: Your future comes first.
>
> As Moloney explains, "If it comes down to choosing me instead of your feelings in this relationship, then I always have to choose me because I can't sacrifice how I feel or the things that I want or I need just because it's going to hurt you." It may sound blunt, but it's so much easier than you'd think to put off ending a relationship that's run its course. Dealing with how it might make the other person feel, or even confronting the messiness of conflict in general are sometimes compelling reasons to keep quiet. Trust me when I say avoiding it now will only make it blow up ten times worse than it needs to be. A big regret among the young women I spoke to was not ending something sooner, even though they knew a breakup would be inevitable. The end result? Wasting precious college years while you value not rocking the boat over your emotional development and freedom. Knock it off!
>
> Long story short? You should never be in a relationship you don't want to be in. Just end it, and don't think twice.

On Ghosting

We haven't always had a catchy term for it, but trust me when I say people have been awkwardly ending hookups by ignoring the other person since long before you were born. There is no greater soul-crushing experience than running into someone who saw you naked the night before, prepping a bagel in the dining hall, only for them to look right through you as though you did not exist. It makes you feel small, used, and crazy. You're left there wondering, *What did I do wrong to make you act without even a shred of human decency? I literally just wanted you to acknowledge me as a fellow human that you know!* This is the kind of behavior, so dreaded by young women, that prevents them from asking for even the bare minimum of clarity or parameters on a hookup, lest they be labeled needy. Resist that urge. When this happens, we obviously crave closure, but we can't force every partner to offer it to us. Instead, Moloney suggests, if you find yourself in this altogether sucky position, ask yourself how you're feeling, and answer honestly. If it's intolerable, maybe you've learned something about your boundaries, and you no longer want to invite in the types of hookups that might breed this outcome. It might also give you a kick in the pants to ask for what you want the next time around. You don't have to forgo casual sex, but you can work up the courage to say at the start of your next hookup, "Hey, I'm down to keep this low-key, but if either of us is feeling like we're over it, I'd like us to be up front about it." Anyone who acts like this is a weird thing to ask is not worth the energy of taking off your bra for, full stop!

WHAT IS A "GOOD" RELATIONSHIP, ANYWAY? SELF-AWARENESS 101

I'm of the opinion that the typical college years are not the time to be thinking seriously about marriage or long-term commitment. There is just so much more time for that in the future than I can possibly convey! But it *is* a good time to start thinking about what you might want or need, theoretically, from a long-term partner. Enter clinical psychologist Alexandra H. Solomon, PhD, who teaches a Marriage 101 course at Northwestern University that she describes as being all "about the self in love." So who better to ask how you figure out what you need in a relationship? How *do* you know what you want?

Solomon explains that the key is understanding the link between "Relational Self-Awareness" and "relationship experience." Relational Self-Awareness is "the ability to take a curious stance vis-à-vis yourself," meaning you should understand how past interpersonal experiences have shaped how you function in relationships now.[1] It also involves understanding and naming your emotions rather than just acting them out, and being able to hear feedback about yourself openly. The more relationally self-aware you are, the easier it may be to identify a compatible partner. Through this process, you can know something about yourself (e.g., "I'm an older sibling so I love to nurture and protect"), and then come to find that in practice things are much different (e.g., "I am smothering my partner by trying to fix all their problems"). As Solomon says, "The insights are one thing, but then living it and honing it and letting the experience of loving and being loved shift us," is another. That's the connection between Relational Self-Awareness and relationship experience: Knowing yourself well can give you a heads-up about issues that may present in a relationship, and the lived experience of a relationship can teach you even more about who you are and how you act with others.

Knowing that you need both experiences, but that only one can be practiced without a partner, how do you become more relationally self-aware? Solomon thrilled me when she said a book like this one helps. That's because knowledge acquisition is key. Tools like diagrams of the human anatomy, scripts for moments of conflict, and sample language to talk to your partner about pleasure and concern can give you a framework to help you make sense of what you're experiencing, Solomon says. Then there are what she likes to call "Fucking Growth Opportunities," or FGOs,[2] that is, moments of conflict that teach us something. It's important to come at what we might consider a mistake with a lot of self-compassion. If we interrogate those moments with empathy, instead of being mad at ourselves for not having it all figured out, then we have an opportunity to learn and grow. If you're too focused on the mistake itself, you'll miss the chance to get something out of it.

Another strategy to guide you on the path to Relational Self-Awareness and discerning what you actually want from partnerships is breaking your motivations down into love-guided choices or fear-driven choices.[3] If you're deciding to have sex with someone, Solomon explains, giving a love-guided "yes" to a question would be because you really want to, because you're curious about it, and so on. A love-guided "no" would be because you're just not ready yet, or not interested. A fear-driven "yes" would be because you're nervous they'll break up with you if you don't. A fear-driven "no" would be because you want to but you're afraid of getting slut-shamed or catching feelings. This is an incredibly powerful tool to better understand your decisions and why you're reacting the way you are both in and out of relationships.

> **"Fucking growth opportunities" are moments of conflict that teach us something.**

The Ins and Outs of Healthy Relationships

How can you recognize the key signs of a healthy relationship? Try what I'm calling the eggshell test. Ideally, according to Solomon, you don't want to feel like you're walking on eggshells around your partner, that you have to tread carefully because any wrong move could make the whole thing crumble. If you *do* have that feeling, how you handle it matters. Say you're experiencing that trepidation. Approach your partner and tell them so. If they react with concern that you're feeling this way, you can sit down together to try and figure out what's going on. Maybe it's a feeling that's totally in your head, or maybe your partner is acting in a way that's causing you to feel this way, but the key is to have an open mind about figuring out what this feeling is telling you about the relationship. If they refuse to talk about your feelings or consistently invalidate them, that's a bad omen. "The sign of a healthy relationship is not whether or not there's conflict or whether or not everyone feels comfortable all the time. It's the degree to which we can meet the experiences we're having with curiosity," Solomon explains. AKA, passing the eggshell test.

Then there are noted psychologist and relationship researcher Dr. John Gottman's Four Horsemen: four qualities that spell disaster for relationship health. Criticism, where we constantly attack our partner's character. Contempt, where we treat our partners with scorn and disrespect, ridiculing them with sarcasm and cruelty. Defensiveness, where we refuse to take responsibility for our actions and shift blame back to our partner. And stonewalling, where we shut down and withdraw from our partner.[4] This doesn't mean that one or two instances of these behaviors means the relationship is doomed, but a relationship with a pattern of these conflict styles and no attempt to work on them would be profoundly unhealthy. Dr. Solomon, who teaches Gottman's work in her course, explains why conflict itself isn't the problem: "The people we love matter to us, so it's easy to get upset. So the question is not whether or not we get upset, it is what do we do when that happens?"

You also want to be on the lookout for patterns of deceit. One or two incidents, if they can be met with curiosity and empathy like in the eggshell test, might be no big deal, and is, in fact, a learning opportunity for you both. But a pattern with no communication around it does not make for a healthy relationship. Take Harper, a junior who goes to school in upstate New York. When Harper was a freshman, she was dating a guy she never felt totally secure with. She didn't feel like their communication was great, and sometimes felt like he wasn't that interested in her sexually. On a long drive to his brother's wedding, Harper saw her boyfriend's phone light up with a bunch of flirty emojis. She knew it was wrong to snoop, but when they stopped for gas she looked through his phone and saw a text conversation with a number she didn't know, and lots of naked photos. When she confronted him about it, he told her it was a cam girl porn service he pays for and that he wasn't cheating. Harper isn't naive; she knows tons of people look at porn, and that in and of itself does not constitute a betrayal. But she felt really uneasy about the fact that he was developing this intimate-feeling relationship with one or two specific models, rather than just browsing the internet. Harper was hurt that he didn't seem interested in having sex with her, but he'd pay to see other women naked. She asked him how he thought this could be okay without talking to her first and he didn't have an answer. She put her headphones on for the rest of the drive and they settled into a cold, tense silence. That night, they went to his brother's rehearsal dinner and Harper pretended everything was fine. They went back and forth about it later that night, but ultimately she dropped it. "I had a self-esteem issue where I was like, 'I need him. I need this person who I think wants me, who wants me enough to say I'm their girlfriend. I'm gonna hold on to that, and I'll forgive him and believe that this is just porn and move past it,'" Harper tells me.

But it's hard to move past something that just keeps happening. A few months later, they were attending Harper's sister's wedding (they have bad luck with weddings!) when her boyfriend's phone lit up, alerting her to yet another conflict. A girl's name popped up on his screen and Harper asked him who he was texting with. He explained that it was his friend's fiancée, who his friend thought was cheating on him. So, his friend group decided that Harper's boyfriend should start chatting her up, to prove that she was a cheater. Harper was incredulous. Essentially, he was flirting with this girl as bait to prove some past alleged infidelity. Again, she found herself asking, how could you think this is okay? Isn't there someone without a girlfriend who could be doing this? He tried to get other wedding guests on his side, to insist this was no big deal, but no one agreed. The part that hurt Harper is that he so readily volunteered and didn't discuss it with her first. But she was scared to be alone and didn't break up with him, even now that a pattern had emerged. She started picking fights and pushing him away, and eventually they broke things off a few months later.

Eggshells, deceit, and the four horsemen aren't the only ways to tell if you're in an unhealthy relationship, but if you notice an upsetting pattern of behavior, it's never a bad idea to slow down and ask yourself: Do I want to be stuck in this loop forever?

Healthy Communication

One predictor of a satisfying relationship is communication skills.[5] To get a better sense of what "happy" communication styles look like, we turn again to the work of John Gottman, PhD, which suggests that there are three types of communication styles among happy couples: conflict avoidant, volatile, and validating.[6] Conflict-avoidant couples aren't passive-aggressive, they just genuinely mean "It's fine" when they say "It's fine." They often agree to disagree and have strong boundaries and independence. Volatile couples argue and debate passionately and often, but without mean-spiritedness or contempt—think: makeup sex! Validating couples are what you might think of when two therapists get together. They practice a lot of empathy and make it a point to try and understand and support their partner's point of view. Each of these types of communication styles represents a happy couple.

You might run into some speed bumps when you have two differing styles in one relationship. Someone who is conflict avoidant might struggle with someone who is volatile and really wants to debate every issue. But this doesn't mean you can't have happy, healthy relationships with someone who communicates differently than you. The key is acceptance. No one partner is going to be able to give us everything we need emotionally, mentally, and spiritually. If the relationship is otherwise healthy and happy, focus on what you get from your partner and figure out where you can turn for what you don't. For example, if you're a validating person and your partner isn't, maybe you call up your best friend if you're looking to have an hours-long conversation dissecting your current dilemma with your adviser about your major. It doesn't mean your current partner doesn't support you or care about these issues, it just means that if you want to have a specific interaction with lots of affirmation and follow-up questions, you might need to seek out someone who tends to communicate in those ways.

Then there's learning trust. If you're avoidant, your partner may need to learn to trust you when you say there's nothing wrong. (This might be hard for a validating or volatile communicator who wants to get deeper into "it," even if there's nothing there to discuss!) And it doesn't mean your partner will be incapable of adjusting as necessary, either. Solomon explains that without criticizing, you can "lovingly prompt" your partner with phrases like, "Hey, I need a little bit more from you in this conversation. I just dealt with something really hard and I could use some validation." Taking a step back to look at these styles can give you some useful data about how to approach conflict.

The Five Love Languages

Another helpful tool in the "let's gather some data" chest is The Five Love Languages, developed in the eponymous book by Dr. Gary Chapman. These are five different common ways we might give and receive love. They are: words of affirmation, quality time, receiving gifts, acts of service, and physical touch.[7] If you're trying to figure out which one most represents you, ask yourself, if you're having a crappy day, what would you most want your partner to do: give you a validating pep talk, lie by your side watching a movie and chatting, surprise you with flowers, do those dishes that have been piling up even though it was your turn, or give you a deep massage followed by a cuddle? That's probably not a foolproof quiz, but you get the general idea. You absolutely don't need those styles to align in a couple in order to have a successful relationship. But they can be a useful framework for figuring out your wants and needs. If you're feeling like your partner never shows affection, it could just be that they're showing it in ways that you don't perceive as love. After all, bringing notes from your Bio lab to your dorm because you were sick and missed class doesn't exactly feel sexy. But examining these affection styles together can help couples understand there's no such thing as a hierarchy when it comes to showing love.

Love and Commitment

How do you know you're in love? That's a loaded question, no doubt. Some of us, Solomon explains, fall in love. Others step quite cautiously. The expression itself can lead those of us who didn't immediately see fireworks to assume we're doing it wrong, or to doubt our feelings. There's no handy checklist I can give you for this one. Being in love is going to look different for everyone. But Solomon likes to think of it as wanting to make choices that elevate and support another person. That doesn't mean unconditional support at the expense of you, though.

Love means wanting to cheer for each other, wanting to be a positive part of how each of you grow, develop, and meet your goals. That's a key feature to keep in mind when you're thinking about longer-term commitments, or even marriage. Ask yourself: Do I feel like this relationship is resilient enough to change and grow with me? How does this relationship support my intellectual and emotional development? Do I have to dim my light to make sure my partner isn't threatened by me?

Who you are and what you need can and will change from your twenties to your thirties, fifties, and beyond. Before making any serious commitments, you'll want to feel sure that the partnership you're in can adapt as you do. There are a lot of myths about healthy long-term relationships. Contrary to popular belief, yes, you'll fight. You won't always feel like things are easy. You'll get nostalgic for past relationships. You won't always want to have sex. But with a foundation of honesty, a willingness to hear each other out, an intrinsic drive to support each other, and a commitment to communicating as effectively as you can, you'll have a good clue that you've found something special.

eeee

Love and relationships are a beautiful, tangly, complicated mess. I felt that most keenly right after I got engaged. We had just gotten home from an Alka-Seltzer-level indulgent dinner when I started to loosen the straps on my heels. My toes cautiously uncurled with relief, a sure sign to my boyfriend that I would be braless and sweatpants-clad in a mere matter of seconds. "Wait!" he shouted from the other room. "Don't put pajamas on yet!"

Pumps in hand, I turned around and saw him waiting hesitantly, one knee grazing the hardwood floor of our living room. Just a few moments later, we were engaged.

Like most people who are sort of expecting their partner to propose (and my god, I hope you are expecting it—the decision to marry shouldn't be a surprise), I was thrilled when mine finally did. I say "finally" not in some "I had a gaping, existential void that only a shiny rock can fill!" way, but more in the "I'd really like to cease wondering when this thing that I'm vaguely anticipating will be over, so I can stop thinking about it" kind of way. But then again, I've always been romantic like that.

After my future husband shakily rose up from the floor and we hugged and I cried just a little, I had a proposal of my own. "How would you feel if we, like . . . didn't tell anyone about this for a while?" I asked. He agreed faster than he's ever agreed to anything. We were headed off to Hawaii the next day, and a vacation seemed like the perfect time to get some space and really enjoy our engagement without having to explain to anyone that no, we hadn't picked a date yet, and no, I didn't know what my "colors" would be.

And it worked! We had initially planned to call our parents and in-dulge their kvelling halfway through the trip but ultimately pushed it back to when we returned. I didn't want to spend one of our precious beach days sitting on my phone, refreshing the likes on an engagement announcement on Instagram. (I know myself, that is exactly what I would have done.) We proceeded to eat fish tacos, snorkel, and do all manner of beach-vacation things.

And then we got home. On the morning we had agreed to call our loved ones with our news, I woke up feeling like I was in a straitjacket. I willed my lungs to expand but instead drew in only sharp, shallow breaths. Suddenly, the idea of picking up the phone filled me with equal parts dread and nausea.

Immobilized by the realization that once we told people, our engage-ment would finally be "real," I felt the apprehension set in. And although it was one of the most joyous milestones of my life to date, lying in bed on that Saturday morning, I began to piece together why I felt so sad. The truth is, I knew I'd miss certain aspects of my single life. I'd miss that feeling of dabbing on sultry perfume and sauntering off to a bar with the delicious feeling that anything might happen. I'd miss pulling myself out of a stranger's bed, hailing a cab at 4 AM, and pouring myself back into my own. I'd miss the egg sandwich I'd order around 1 PM the day to restore my depleted calories and soak up the vodka sodas.

Why did it feel like a betrayal to my new fiancé, even to myself, just to admit that? I don't necessarily want to be doing those things now. I am older, my tolerance for alcohol has diminished, and I'll be frank: I feel absolutely no pull toward an open relationship. I just needed to feel that honoring my nostalgia for those moments wasn't a sign my marriage was doomed.

While I'd been off on vacation, sipping mojitos and working on my sunburn, all of those normal wedding jitters had been piling up in my subconscious. For a week during our engagement embargo, I didn't have my friends to unleash my nerves on, and in turn bask in the comfort of hearing, "Wow, you've become unhinged. Please come back down to reality in which you are fine and marrying a person you love." Every fear had become so pressurized by the buildup of time that our exciting secret started to feel like an unbearable burden. I was still in bed, stewing in my nerves and what I thought they might mean, when I started to cry.

"This is so big," I told him. "I'm just scared."

"Me, too," he said, stroking my hair softly.

His compassion and honesty in the face of my doubts made the knot in my stomach begin to loosen. We made one call, and then another. Looser still. But I didn't really feel better until I called one of my closest friends. I rattled the saga off to her: I had just gotten engaged, and I was a little scared. Was I doing this wrong already?

Hearing it all out loud gave me the solace I needed. I needed to be kinder myself, my friend reminded me. This was never about doubting whether I should marry my partner. I've known for years I wanted to. He's funny, kind, and makes my life exciting and unpredictable in all the best ways.

It was about the nature of choices.

To go on a date with someone is a choice. To go to bed with them, another. To marry them, an even bigger one. And to actively love them with intention and empathy is a choice you'll have to keep making every day. Any choice, even the most blissful ones, can come at the expense of giving up something else. Another person, another alternate timeline your life could have taken, another job you didn't get or trip you didn't book. In its own way, going through any life transition requires mourning for the past version of you that's left behind. There's nothing wrong with feeling a little sad at a time the world is telling you to smile. It doesn't mean you're making a mistake or not truly in love; it simply means that you've had wonderful memories worth preserving. That you can hold two conflicting feelings in your hand without feeling compelled to crush one or the other out of sheer panic. It means that you're human.

I couldn't outrun my engagement anxiety, or leave it on a beach in Hawaii. So I did something different. I felt my nerves, absolved myself of my fears, and delighted in the person who loves me through them all. I think that's a pretty good way to take the next step in any relationship.

Congrats, Grad!

Learning about yourself—your wants and needs, your likes and dislikes, your body and its quirks—is like earning a degree unto itself. And it's far more important than just about any academic achievement you'll ever make (don't tell your parents). It's hard work, and you should be proud that you've started putting in the thought and effort to figure it out. This work is messy. There's a reason this book is full of sound advice and a heaping handful of my own mistakes. I wrote candidly about those mistakes not so that you can avoid them, but so that you'll have strategies and guidance to course correct for the many unique blunders you'll make all on your own.

And that's a good thing.

I would love to send you off into the world so prepared, so self-aware that you never have a single sexual experience that's anything less than stellar. But I don't have to tell you that's near impossible, because sometimes you can't figure out what you like without figuring out what you don't. Sometimes people who seem to have your best interests at heart are more interested in breaking it than caring for it. And sometimes you'll do stupid things with people you care about because you didn't know any better. All of that is okay, especially if you can learn to take the pressure and judgment off yourself when something doesn't go the way you planned. If you're holding on to guilt about a moment when you "should have known better," it's time to let it go.

As you move excitedly, tentatively, or fearfully through these transitional years of your life, hold fast to a deep-seated belief that you are entitled to 100 percent of your intimate desires and beholden to no one else's. If that's the one guiding principle you carry forward with you, from graduation and beyond, you're going to be just fine.

Notes

Chapter 1

1. Jennifer L. Kerpelman, et al., "Engagement in Risky Sexual Behavior: Adolescents' Perceptions of Self and the Parent–Child Relationship Matter," *Youth & Society* 48, no. 1 (March 3, 2013): 101–25.

2. Christina Maxouris and Saeed Ahmed, "Only These 8 States Require Sex Education Classes to Mention Consent," CNN, September 29, 2018.

3. "Less Than Half of People Think It's OK to Withdraw Sexual Consent If They're Already Naked," Family Planning Association, September 2018, fpa.org.uk/less-than-half-of-people-think-its-ok-to-withdraw-sexual-consent-if-theyre-already-naked.

Chapter 2

1. "Sexually Transmitted Infections Prevalence, Incidence, and Cost Estimates in the United States," Centers for Disease Control and Prevention (CDC), February 18, 2021, cdc.gov/std/statistics/prevalence-incidence-cost-2020.htm.

2. Hannah Smothers, "7 Dangerous Sex Myths Teens Still Learn in American Classrooms," *Cosmopolitan*, November 2, 2018.

3. Ibid.

4. "STDs & Infertility," CDC, October 30, 2013, cdc.gov/std/infertility/default.htm.

5. Dan Xiao, et al., "Effects of a Short-Term Mass-Media Campaign Against Smoking," *The Lancet* 382, no. 9909 (December 14, 2013): 1964–66.

6. "New CDC Report: STDs Continue to Rise in the U.S.," CDC, October 8, 2019, cdc.gov/nchhstp/newsroom/2019/2018-STD-surveillance-report-press-release.html.

7. "Herpes—STI Treatment Guidelines," CDC, July 22, 2021, cdc.gov/std/treatment-guidelines/herpes.htm.

8. "Genital Herpes—CDC Fact Sheet," CDC, August 28, 2017, cdc.gov/std/herpes/stdfact-herpes.htm.

9. "How HIV Impacts LGBTQ+ People," Human Rights Campaign, February 2017, hrc.org/resources/hrc-issue-brief-hiv-aids-and-the-lgbt-community.

Chapter 3

1. Betsy Foxman, et al., "Health Behavior and Urinary Tract Infection in College-Aged Women," *Journal of Clinical Epidemiology* 43, no. 4 (Winter 1990).

2. Antonia Abbey, PhD, "Alcohol-Related Sexual Assault: A Common Problem Among College Students." *Journal of Studies on Alcohol*, Suppl. 14 (2002).

3. "Data Report Spring 2019," American College Health Association (ACHA), National College Health Assessment, acha.org/documents/ncha/NCHA-II_SPRING_2019_UNDERGRADUATE_REFERENCE_GROUP_DATA_REPORT.pdf.

4. Ibid.

5. Sandra A. Brown, et al., "A Developmental Perspective on Alcohol and Youths 16 to 20 Years of Age," *Pediatrics* 121, Suppl. 4 (April 2008): 30–32.

Chapter 4

1. C. Abma, PhD, et al., "Sexual Activity and Contraceptive Use Among Teenagers in the United States, 2011–2015," National Health Statistics Reports, no. 104, (June 2017): 6.

2. Christopher Ingraham, "The Share of Americans Not Having Sex Has Reached a Record High," *The Washington Post*, March 29, 2019.

3. Ali Drucker, "The Secrets To to Great Sex If You Have Anxiety," HuffPost, May 31, 2019.

4. Ali Drucker, "The Secrets to Great Sex If You Have Anxiety," HuffPost, May 31, 2019.

5. "Data Report Spring 2019," ACHA, op. cit.

6. Justin R. Garcia, et al., "Sexual Hookup Culture: A Review," *Review of General Psychology* 16, no. 2 (June 2012): 36.

Chapter 5

1. E. Sandra Byers, "Beyond the *Birds and the Bees* and *Was It Good for You?*: Thirty Years of Research on Sexual Communication," *Canadian Psychology* 52, no. 1 (2011): 20–28.

2. Charlene L. Muehlenhard and Sheena K. Shippee, "Men's and Women's Reports of Pretending Orgasm," *The Journal of Sex Research* 47, no. 6 (2010): 9–10.

Chapter 6

1. "2018 LGBTQ Youth Report," Human Rights Campaign (HRC), 2018, assets2.hrc.org/files/assets/resources/2018-YouthReport-0514-Final.pdf.

2. "Preventing Suicide: Facts About Suicide," The Trevor Project, thetrevorproject.org/resources/preventing-suicide/facts-about-suicide.

3. "2018 LGBTQ Youth Report," HRC, op. cit.

4. "Transgender Identity and Experiences of Violence Victimization, Substance Use, Suicide Risk, and Sexual Risk Behaviors Among High School Students—19 States and Large Urban School Districts, 2017," CDC Morbidity and Mortality Weekly Report, January 25, 2019, cdc.gov/mmwr/volumes/68/wr/mm6803a3.htm.

5. Ronnie Cohen, "After Men, Lesbians Report the Most Orgasms During Sex," *Reuters*, August 25, 2014, reuters.com/article/us-orgasm-rates-idUSKBN0GP1CM20140825.

6. James Sorensen, et al., "Evaluation and Treatment of Female Sexual Pain: A Clinical Review," *Cureus* 10, no. 3 (March 27, 2018).

Chapter 7

1. Ariel Shensa, et al., "Social Media Use and Depression and Anxiety Symptoms: A Cluster Analysis," *American Journal of Health Behavior* 42, no. 2 (March 2018): 116–28.

2. Marijke Naezer and Jessica Ringrose, "Adventure, Intimacy, Identity and Knowledge: Exploring How Social Media Are Shaping and Transforming Youth Sexuality," in *The Cambridge Handbook of Sexual Development: Childhood and Adolescence*, Sharon Lamb, ed. (Cambridge University Press, 2018): 419–39.

3. Camille Mori, et al., "The Prevalence of Sexting Behaviors Among Emerging Adults: A Meta-Analysis," *Archives of Sexual Behavior* 49 (February 2020): 1103–19.

4. Amanda Lenhart, et al., "Nonconsensual Image Sharing: One in 25 Americans Has Benn a Victim of 'Revenge Porn,'" Data & Society Research Institute, Center for Innovative Public Health Research, December 13, 2016, datasociety.net/pubs/oh/Nonconsensual_Image_Sharing_2016.pdf.

Chapter 8

1. R. P. Auerbach, et al., "WHO World Mental Health Surveys International College Student Project: Prevalence and Distribution of Mental Disorders," *Journal of Abnormal Psychology* 127, no. 7 (2018): 623–38.

2. "Frequently Asked Questions about College Student Mental Health Data and Statistics," The Healthy Minds Network, April 2019, healthymindsnetwork.org/wp-content/uploads/2019/04/FAQs-about-Student-Mental-Health-Data-and-Statistics_FINAL.pdf.

3. "Mental Health Disorders in Adolescents," American College of Obstetricians and Gynecologists, 2020, acog.org/clinical/clinical-guidance/committee-opinion/articles/2017/07/mental-health-disorders-in-adolescents.

4. Sarah Ketchen Lipson, PhD, et al., "Increased Rates of Mental Health Service Utilization by U.S. College Students: 10-Year Population-Level Trends (2007–2017)," *Psychiatric Services* 70, no. 1 (January 2019): 60–63.

5. "Meet Gen Z: Gun Violence, Immigration, Sexual Harassment Stressing America's Youngest Adults; Most Likely to Report Poor Mental Health," American Psychological Association, Stress in America Survey, 2018, apa.org/news/press/releases/stress/2018/stress-gen-z.pdf.

6. "2018 LGBTQ Youth Report" Human Rights Campaign, 2018, assets2.hrc.org/files/assets/resources/2018-YouthReport-0514-Final.pdf.

7. Edward Chesney, et al., "Risks of All Cause and Suicide Mortality in Mental Disorders: A Meta Review," *World Psychiatry* 13, no. 2 (June 2014): 153–60.

8. "Eating Disorders on the College Campus: A National Survey of Programs and Resources," National Eating Disorders Association, February 2013, nationaleatingdisorders.org/sites/default/files/CollegeSurvey/CollegiateSurveyProject.pdf.

9. Ibid.

Chapter 9

1. Sara Lindberg, "How to Avoid Getting a UTI After Sex," *Healthline*, November 19, 2019, healthline.com/health/uti-after-sex#_noHeaderPrefixedContent.

2. "The Talk: How Adults Can Promote Young People's Healthy Relationships and Prevent Misogyny and Sexual Harassment," Making Caring Common Project, Harvard Graduate School of Education, May 2017, mcc.gse.harvard.edu/reports/the-talk.

3. "Half of All Teens Feel Uncomfortable Talking to Their Parents About Sex While Only 19 Percent of Parents Feel the Same, New Survey Shows," Planned Parenthood, January 30, 2014, plannedparenthood.org/about-us/newsroom/press-releases/half-all-teens-feel-uncomfortable-talking-their-parents-about-sex-while-only-19-percent-parents.

4. "The Talk: How Adults Can Promote Young People's Healthy Relationships and Prevent Misogyny and Sexual Harassment," Making Caring Common Project, Harvard Graduate School of Education, May 2017, mcc.gse.harvard.edu/reports/the-talk.

Chapter 10

1. "Campus Sexual Violence: Statistics," RAINN, https://rainn.org/statistics/campus-sexual-violence.

2. "Statistics," Know Your IX, knowyourix.org/issues/statistics.

3. David Cantor, et al., "Report on the AAU Campus Climate Survey on Sexual Assault and Misconduct," The Association of American Universities, January 17, 2020, aau.edu/sites/default/files/AAU-Files/Key-Issues/Campus-Safety/Revised%20Aggregate%20report%20%20and%20appendices%201-7_(01-16-2020_FINAL).pdf.

4. Ibid.

5. "Full Report of the Prevalence, Incidence, and Consequences of Violence Against Women," Findings from the National Violence Against Women Survey, November 2000, ojp.gov/pdffiles1/nij/183781.pdf.

6. "What Is a Rape Kit and Rape Kit Exam?," End the Backlog, endthebacklog.org/information-survivors-dna-and-rape-kit-evidence/what-rape-kit-and-rape-kit-exam.

7. Charlene Y. Senn, PhD, et al., "Efficacy of a Sexual Assault Resistance Program for University Women," *New England Journal of Medicine* (June 11, 2015).

8. "Our Whole Lives: Lifespan Sexuality Education," Unitarian Universalist Association, uua.org/re/owl.

Chapter 11

1. Alexandra H. Solomon, PhD, *Loving Bravely: Twenty Lessons of Self-Discovery to Help You Get the Love You Want* (Oakland, CA: New Harbinger Publications, 2017), 2.

2. ———, *Taking Sexy Back: How to Own Your Sexuality and Create the Relationships You Want* (Oakland, CA: New Harbinger Publications, 2020).

3. ———, *Relational Self-Awareness: The Key to Navigating Modern Love*, Ted Talk, June 2019, San Juan Islands, Washington, ted.com/talks/alexandra_solomon_relational_self_awareness_the_key_to_navigating_modern_love.

4. Ellie Lisitsa, "The Four Horsemen: Criticism, Contempt, Defensiveness, and Stonewalling," *Gottman Institute Blog*, April 23, 2013, gottman.com/blog/the-four-horsemen-recognizing-criticism-contempt-defensiveness-and-stonewalling.

5. Sine Eğeci and Tülin Gençöz, "Factors Associated with Relationship Satisfaction: Importance of Communication Skills," *Contemporary Family Therapy* 28 (2006): 383–91.

6. John Gottman, PhD, "The 5 Types of Couples," *Gottman Institute Blog*, November 22, 2014, gottman.com/blog/the-5-couple-types.

7. *The Five Love Languages*, Wikipedia, February 20, 2021, en.wikipedia.org/wiki/The_Five_Love_Languages.

Acknowledgments

I am profoundly grateful to have so many people's efforts to acknowledge.

To my parents, Robin and Bruce: everything I am is because of you. Your endless well of love and support gave me my voice. I will always try to use it to make you proud. I'm sorry I didn't dedicate this book to you, but considering the subject matter, it would have been a little weird. I love you both.

To my husband, Jesse: thank you for creating the space I needed to turn a dream into reality. I will never forget how remarkably encouraging you were about a book that detailed my past sex life. Just one of the countless reasons why you forever have my heart.

To my sister, Lacey, for letting me borrow so many of your clothes in college.

To my agents, Todd Shuster and Justin Brouckaert, for being the first to believe in and champion this project.

To my editor, Batya Rosenblum, for your steadfast and thoughtful work making this book shine. If you weren't here to slash my unnecessary use of the word "basically," push me to be more precise, and share my big dreams for this project, I'd be lost.

To my friends: because of you, college wasn't just a place, it was a home.

To everyone who lent their time, expertise, and deeply personal stories to bring this book to life: thank you, thank you, thank you. This work could not exist without you.

About the Author

ALI DRUCKER is a freelance writer based in Los Angeles who covers sexual health and pop culture. She lives with her husband, temperamental cat, and moderately well-behaved dog. You can find her work in *The New York Times*, *New York* magazine, HuffPost, Refinery29, and more. She previously served as the senior sex and relationships senior editor at *Maxim* and *Cosmo*. When she's not interviewing people about their sex lives, Ali enjoys loading up on SPF and going to the beach, taking easy hikes, and snuggling with her pets while watching old episodes of shows she's seen a million times on Netflix.

alidrucker.com | 🐦 📷 ali_drucker